Stillness in Motion: The Campfire Guide to Traditional Vinyasa Yoga

Stillness in Motion: The Campfire Guide to Traditional Vinyasa Yoga

Francis Williams

Copyright Page

Stillness in Motion: The Campfire Guide to Traditional Vinyasa Yoga
© 2025 Francis Williams
All rights reserved.

Publisher:
Quite Frank Educational Services
Richmond, BC, Canada

Cover design by the author.
Printed in the United States of America.

First Edition: 2025
ISBN: 978-1-997668-62-6

Publisher's Note

This book represents the author's independent research and reflection. The opinions expressed are those of the author and do not necessarily reflect the views of Quite Frank Educational Services or any affiliated organization.

Stillness in Motion:
The Campfire Guide to Traditional Vinyasa Yoga

Table of Contents

"You do not have to seek freedom in a different land, for it exists with your own body, heart, mind, and soul."

~ B.K.S. Iyengar

"The success of Yoga does not lie in the ability to perform postures, but in how it positively changes the way we live our life and our relationships."

~ T.K.V. Desikachar

"Yoga is the journey of the self, through the self, to the self."

~ The Bhagavad Gītā

"Be yourself; everyone else is already taken."

~ Oscar Wilde

"Inhale the future, exhale the past."

~ Author Unknown (widely quoted in yoga circles and workshops)

"Peace comes from within. Do not seek it without."

~ The Buddha

Disclaimer

The material presented in *Stillness in Motion: The Campfire Guide to Traditional Vinyasa Yoga* is for informational and educational purposes only. It is not intended to replace professional medical advice, diagnosis, or treatment. Always consult with a qualified healthcare provider before beginning any new exercise, wellness, or breathwork program, especially if you have pre-existing conditions or concerns.

The author and publisher assume no liability for injuries or damages arising from the use or misuse of the information contained in this book. Readers are encouraged to practice with care, respect their own limits, and seek qualified instruction when appropriate.

This book includes humorous anecdotes and metaphors intended for engagement and relatability. These do not diminish the seriousness or sacredness of yoga traditions. Cultural terms, practices, and stories are included with respect to their origins and contexts.

AI Acknowledgement

In addition to traditional research methods, this book's research, editing, and structuring were supported by AI-powered tools. Specifically, large language model systems were used to:

- Organize and summarize source material.
- Suggest narrative flow, metaphors, and stylistic enhancements.
- Assist in drafting, revising, and fact-checking sections.

All final content was reviewed, shaped, and approved by the human author to ensure accuracy, authenticity, and alignment with the intended voice. AI assistance did not replace human authorship or judgment; it acted as a co-creative research and editorial tool.

This acknowledgement is offered in the spirit of transparency and integrity.

Introduction: Welcome to the Flow (or, How I Learned to Love My Breath and Stop Competing with the Guy in Lululemon)

There's a moment in every yoga class — somewhere between your third Chaturanga and your impending existential crisis in Pigeon Pose — when you think, *What am I doing with my life?*

Sometimes that moment passes. Sometimes, it becomes the doorway to something much deeper than just tighter glutes.

Welcome, friend. You've just stumbled into the warm, flickering light of a campfire we've been tending for generations. This book is not a how-to manual filled with pictures of people contorted like artistic pretzels. It's a storytelling adventure through the wild, winding, occasionally sweaty world of Traditional Vinyasa Yoga — a practice that's older than your favorite playlist but somehow more relevant than ever in this age of dopamine notifications and stress-induced jaw clenching.

Let's get one thing out of the way early:

Vinyasa is not just "fast yoga."
It's not just a cardio-fueled, breathy power hour designed to help you "detox" after taco night. That's like saying a pub is just a place to get drunk — technically true but missing the point entirely.

Vinyasa, in its traditional form, is a living philosophy, a moving meditation, and an art form of *placing things in a special way* — not just your limbs, but your breath, your attention, and your intention. It's part poetry, part science, part philosophy, and part "I can't feel my thighs but somehow I feel... peace?"

So, what Is This Book Really About?

This book is your witty, research-backed, chai-sipping, occasionally sarcastic companion through the roots, philosophy, and evolution of Vinyasa yoga. We'll unpack Sanskrit words like we're unboxing old high school mixtapes — reverently, but also with a little side-eye.

We'll journey through ancient texts like the *Yoga Sutras of Patanjali* and the *Bhagavad Gita* — not like monks in a Himalayan cave, but like curious humans trying to make sense of rush-hour traffic, existential dread, and that one guy who breathes really loudly in class (you know the one).

We'll look at the science behind the flow — what your brain's doing during Ujjayi breath, how focus sharpens when you lock your gaze on your big toe, and why a little internal heat (a.k.a. tapas) is better than a double shot of espresso for mental clarity.

And most importantly, we'll tell stories.

Because *Traditional Vinyasa* isn't just something you do on a mat — it's something you feel in your bones, carry in your breath, and use as a secret weapon when your toddler melts down in the cereal aisle or your boss drops a last-minute deadline. It's yoga not as escape, but as engagement. Not as flexibility, but as flow — in life, in movement, in meaning.

But Wait — Is This Book for Me?

Let's do a quick check-in:

- Are you a yoga newbie trying to figure out why everyone keeps saying "namaste" like it's a secret password?

- A long-time practitioner wondering if there's more to Vinyasa than doing 57 variations of Warrior Two?

- A health geek who likes your neuroscience served with a side of Sanskrit and sarcasm?

2

- A spiritual seeker who's mildly allergic to gurus but deeply curious about how movement can become meditation?

- Or maybe you're just here for the jokes and hoping to touch your toes without crying?

If you answered "yes" to any of the above, you're in the right place.

This book isn't about becoming more enlightened than your neighbor. It's about *belonging* — to your body, your breath, and a tradition that invites you to show up, every day, as your weird and wonderful self.

A Note on Style (or Why We Talk About Bandhas Like Family Members)

You'll notice a few things as you flip through these pages:

- We talk about philosophy the way your uncle tells ghost stories — with reverence, but also the occasional fart joke.

- We use campfires, pubs, kitchens, and old friends as metaphors for abstract yogic ideas, because metaphysics is more fun when snacks are involved.

- We do research, but we explain it like your favorite high school teacher who made mitochondria feel like a Marvel character.

- We sprinkle in humor breaks — short quips, metaphors, or rants — so your brain gets a stretch too.

What You'll Walk Away With

By the end of this book, you'll have a deep understanding of:

- What Traditional Vinyasa Yoga *actually* is (hint: it's not a yoga playlist on Spotify)

- How ancient wisdom and modern science agree on more than you'd think

- Why breath is more powerful than your overachieving inner critic

- How to build sequences like a wise old yoga grandma

- And most importantly — how to find stillness even when life won't stop moving

Because let's be real: the world isn't slowing down anytime soon. But you can.

One breath, one movement, one lovingly placed intention at a time.

Now grab a blanket, unroll your mat, pour some metaphorical tea, and settle in.

We've got stories to tell — and you're part of the tribe now.

Chapter 1: The Mat, the Myth, the Vinyasa — How We Got Here

In which yoga history is rewritten like a Netflix docuseries and Sanskrit is explained using sandwiches.

Picture this: You walk into your first "Vinyasa Flow" class. The teacher is playing ambient sitar music. There's a guy in the corner warming up like he's auditioning for Cirque du Soleil. And your mat — freshly unrolled, vaguely judgmental — stares back at you like, *Well?*

Five minutes in, you're flailing through a series of sun salutations that feel more like synchronized swimming with no water and a suspicious amount of sweating. The teacher says something about your "Ujjayi breath," and you're wondering if that's a Pokemon or a yoga tax write-off.

Welcome, my friend, to the glorious, confusing, wildly misrepresented world of Vinyasa Yoga.

But don't worry — you're not alone in this labyrinth of flowy sequences, Sanskrit words, and existential quadriceps cramping. Most of us entered Vinyasa thinking it was a trendy workout with a side of deep breathing. Turns out, it's a centuries-old conversation between body and breath, lineage and innovation, discipline and creativity. It's ancient tradition reinvented for people like us — who get anxious opening emails and forget what they walked into the kitchen for.

So how did we get here?

Vinyasa: Not Just a Fancy Way to Say "Yoga with Movement"

Let's start with the word itself: Vinyāsa. Sounds mystical, right? Like something you might whisper to open a secret door in a temple full of bendy monks. But here's where it gets delightfully nerdy.

In Sanskrit, "vi" means "in a special way," and "nyāsa" means "to place." So literally, vinyāsa = to place something in a special way.

Cue the first metaphor of many:

If you're making a sandwich — and you slap lettuce, peanut butter, and pickles together without intention — that's lunch.

But if you *place* each ingredient with thought, layering textures, balancing flavors, maybe toasting the bread just so... that's a Vinyasa sandwich.

In yoga terms, that could mean the sequencing of poses. But it also refers to how you place your breath, your attention, your effort. It's not just about *what* you do — it's about *how* and *why* you do it.

A Brief, Highly Selective History of Vinyasa (Told Like a Campfire Story)

Let's time-travel a bit, shall we?

Back in ancient India, long before boutique yoga studios and gluten-free mats, "nyāsa" was a sacred ritual. Practitioners would place mantras — sacred sound formulas — onto parts of the body. It was about invoking divine energy, literally installing it into the self. Kind of like a metaphysical body tattoo, minus the needles and regret.

This wasn't "flow yoga" in the modern sense. It was spiritual tech.

Fast-forward a few millennia, and a brilliant, mustachioed scholar named Sri T. Krishnamacharya comes along in the early 20th century. He's a Sanskrit master, healer, and yogi who believed that yoga wasn't one-size-fits-all. Instead of forcing students into rigid systems, he tailored sequences to the individual — a radical idea in a world of cookie-cutter spirituality.

He emphasized breath-synchronized movement, turning the transitions *between* poses into sacred, intentional actions — not just filler. This wasn't aerobics in Sanskrit; it was meditation in motion. He called it Vinyasa Krama — step-by-step, intelligent progression.

Now Krishnamacharya had a few famous students. You may have heard of them:

- **Pattabhi Jois**: turned Vinyasa into Ashtanga — strict series, sweat, discipline, rinse, repeat.

- **B.K.S. Iyengar**: slowed it down, added props, said "alignment or bust."

- **T.K.V. Desikachar**: Krishnamacharya's son, who said, "Let's customize it for *you*."

They all interpreted Vinyasa differently — and that's where the fun (and chaos) begins.

From Mysore Palace to Your Local Yoga Studio

What happened next was like yoga's version of the Beatles going solo. Pattabhi Jois's *Ashtanga Vinyasa* was intense, rhythmic, and beautifully structured — like jazz played in six prescribed series. No improvising. No skipping Chaturanga. (Seriously, they'd know.)

Then came the Vinyasa remix:

Western teachers took the breath-and-movement concept and added playlists, creative transitions, and the occasional interpretive dance moment. *Flow yoga* was born — flexible, expressive, sometimes rebellious.

And suddenly, *Vinyasa* became a buzzword. It showed up in gyms, retreats, apps, and — God help us — goat yoga.

But underneath all the branding, the essence remained:

Place breath and movement with intention.

Move like it matters.

Feel every transition like it's the whole point — not just the route to a fancier pose.

Wait — So Is Vinyasa Traditional or Modern?

Both.
That's the twist.

Traditional Vinyasa isn't ancient in its *form* — it didn't drop fully-formed from the Vedas like a yoga instruction manual. But its principles are rooted in deep, classical yogic ideas:

- Meditation through motion (Yoga Sutras)

- Discipline and purification (Hatha Yoga)

- Skillful action without attachment to results (Bhagavad Gītā)

It's like a recipe passed down through generations — everyone adds their own spice, but the soul of the dish stays the same.

Humor Break: Sanskrit Words You Can Say with Confidence (and Maybe a Smile)

- **Ujjayi** – Sounds like a dragon doing calming breaths. Means "victorious breath." Use it when someone cuts you off in traffic.

- **Bandha** – No, not a music group. These are energy locks. Your pelvic floor is basically the bouncer at the nightclub of your soul.

- **Drishti** – The gaze point. Like giving your eyeballs a purpose other than watching yoga pants.

Campfire Takeaway: Where You Place Yourself Matters

Vinyasa isn't about how fancy your pose is — it's about how present you are when you place it.

It's a dance between tradition and creativity, discipline and play. It invites us to show up with all our messiness and say, "Okay, breath — let's move together."

So, the next time you roll out your mat, remember:

You're stepping into a living story.
One that started with ancient mantras and continues every time someone inhales into Upward Dog like they mean it.

You're not just "doing yoga."
You're placing yourself in a special way — breath by breath, step by step, even if you fall out of Tree Pose every single time.

And that, dear reader, is the most traditional thing you can do.

Chapter 2: "To Place in a Special Way": Sanskrit, Sandwiches, and Sequencing

In which we learn that ancient language, when decoded correctly, is kind of like assembling IKEA furniture—satisfying, meaningful, and occasionally infuriating.

Let's begin with a confession: I once thought "Vinyasa" was a brand of yoga pants. True story. I imagined it printed in italic font across the rear of some eco-conscious leggings, maybe with a matching tote.

Turns out, Vinyasa is not a fashion label — though it *has* launched a thousand flows, playlists, and post-practice smoothies. At its core, it's one of those mystical Sanskrit terms that seems simple... until you actually try to explain it without sounding like a yoga fortune cookie.

So, let's break it down. Slowly. Carefully. Like a Sun Salutation taught to your skeptical uncle at a family barbecue.

Deconstructing the Word "Vinyāsa" (With Help From a Sandwich)

Sanskrit has a way of being both poetic and specific — like the language equivalent of a gourmet chef who can also assemble IKEA furniture without crying.

"Vinyāsa" is a compound word.

- "Vi" = *in a special way, apart,* or *with distinction.*

- "Nyāsa" = *to place, to set down, to install.*

Put them together and you get: "to place in a special way."

Sounds poetic, right? But here's where things get tasty. Let's revisit our first recurring motif:

The Vinyasa Sandwich Analogy™

Imagine you're making another sandwich. If you just fling cheese, tomato, and bread together in a chaotic heap, you've got calories, sure — but you don't have lunch.

But if you *place* each ingredient with awareness — toasting the bread just right, layering your fillings, adding a swipe of sauce like you're painting a minimalist masterpiece — well, now you've got a Vinyasa sandwich.

And just like that sandwich, Vinyasa yoga isn't about moving randomly. It's about placing your body, your breath, your intention—each in its own *special way*, like you're building something sacred from the inside out.

From Rituals to Rhythm: Where This All Began

Back in the medieval era — when yoga wasn't about Lululemon, Spotify, or Instagram reels — the word "nyāsa" had a very different job. It was part of tantric ritual, where practitioners would chant mantras and symbolically "place" sacred sounds onto parts of the body.

Think of it as installing spiritual software.
Each body part was a piece of hardware.
Each mantra, a download.

It wasn't about movement — it was about meaning, about mapping divine consciousness onto the human form.

This may seem galaxies away from today's breathy, sweaty Vinyasa classes. But the intention is the through-line. The awareness. The placement — not just of limbs, but of attention. And attention, as modern neuroscience will eagerly tell you, is the currency of consciousness.

The Great 20th-Century Plot Twist

Enter our returning campfire hero: Sri T. Krishnamacharya, the Gandalf of modern yoga. In the early 1900s, Krishnamacharya took the ancient concept of placing mantras on the body... and reimagined it.

He thought: *What if we placed the entire practice — movement, breath, sequencing — in a special way?*

He created a system where you didn't just plop from pose to pose like a yoga ragdoll. Every posture led to the next. Every breath had a job. Even how you moved between poses was part of the experience.

This wasn't just yoga choreography — this was a ritual in motion.

It was called Vinyasa Krama — "the step-by-step progression."
Or, in grandma terms: "Don't skip the sauce and go straight to dessert, sweetheart."

What Makes a Vinyasa Class, Well, Vinyasa?

Modern Vinyasa classes are often freestyle in nature. You may not know what poses are coming. Sometimes, neither does the teacher. (Looking at you, Chad.)

But the best Vinyasa sequences still follow a silent structure — a kind of invisible architecture, grounded in Krishnamacharya's principles of progression. Let's break that down like we're designing a dinner party:

1. Opening Ritual (Appetizer):

Grounding breathwork, intention-setting, or a centering child's pose. This sets the vibe. It's the warm bread before the meal.

2. Warm-Up (Soup Course):

Gentle stretches, shoulder rolls, or cat-cow. Lubricating the joints. Prepping the nervous system.

3. Sun Salutations (First Glass of Wine):

Rhythmic, breath-led movements. They heat you up, activate your cardiovascular system, and trick your brain into thinking you're having fun.

4. The Main Flow (Entrée):

Here's where the sequencing magic happens. Think: standing poses, balances, maybe a juicy peak pose. This is the meat — or tofu — of the practice.

5. Cool Down (Dessert):

Slower floor postures, spinal twists, hip openers. Everything starts to soften. Your mind thinks, *Maybe this wasn't a terrible idea after all.*

6. Savasana (Digestif):

Final rest. Literal stillness. Your reward for not bailing mid-class.

Each phase is intentionally placed — *in a special way* — to move your body from activation to awareness to release. And THAT is the true meaning of Vinyasa.

Humor Break: Why Sequencing Matters (Or, What Happens When It Doesn't)

A poorly sequenced class is like a meal where someone serves cheesecake first, then a flaming curry, then tells you to jog.

Or like getting into Wheel Pose before your spine knows it's out of bed. Or like me attempting a handstand with cold wrists and a hot ego.

Trust me: bad sequencing is the fastest path to injury, grumpiness, and wondering if you're really cut out for this whole "inner peace" thing.

Vinyasa Off the Mat: Sequencing Your Life

Here's where it gets juicy — and a little existential.

Vinyasa Krama isn't just for your mat. It's a life practice. Think about it:

- You don't wake up and launch into a job interview (unless you're very caffeinated and very unemployed).

- You don't start a novel by writing the ending (unless you're George R.R. Martin, and then maybe never write the ending at all).

Life flows better when things are placed with intention — your conversations, your priorities, your responses when your toddler spills oat milk down your shirt.

Traditional Vinyasa teaches us to *sequence our lives* with intelligence.
Step by step.
Stage by stage.
Pose by pose.
Breath by breath.

Campfire Takeaway: Sandwiches, Sequences, and the Sacred Art of Showing Up

When you roll out your mat, you're not just exercising. You're entering a ritual of placement — of layering breath and movement, intention and attention, just like a perfectly made sandwich or a lovingly cooked meal.

Sequencing isn't just smart — it's sacred.
It honors the body's wisdom.
It honors the mind's limits.
And it honors the very heart of yoga: awareness in action.

So next time you're in class, or stuck in traffic, or trying to sequence your words in a difficult conversation — pause.

Ask yourself:

How can I place this moment — my breath, my action — in a special way?

Congratulations.

You've just practiced Vinyasa.

Interlude: Chai, Not Try — A Short Rant About Effortlessness

In which we examine the myth of "letting go," confront our control issues, and spill metaphorical tea all over our ambitions.

Let's talk about *trying*.

You know — that strained, sweaty, overachieving, one-more-pigeon-pose-and-my-hip-will-actually-explode kind of trying.

In yoga, "try" is one of those dangerous little words. Like "just" in emails ("Just checking in…" = I'm already spiraling). Or "organic" in snacks (which somehow justifies eating nine of them).

Every yoga teacher says it at some point:

"Don't try. Just breathe. Let go."

Let go of what exactly? My groceries? My deadlines? My fear of being the only one in class who falls out of Tree Pose like a confused pinecone?

Trying is how we got through high school.

It's how we've survived performance reviews, dating apps, and assembling Swedish furniture using only rage and an Allen wrench.

And then you come to yoga and someone tells you to "let go."

No instructions. No PowerPoint. Just vibes.

Let's Rewind: The Chai Principle

This brings us to what I call the Chai Principle of Effort.

Here's how it works:

When you make chai — real chai, not the boxed stuff that tastes like pumpkin-scented cardboard — you don't just throw spices in a pot and boil the heck out of them while yelling "BE TEA!"

No.

You simmer. You steep.
You add ingredients with patience. You stir with attention.
You *let the flavors unfold* — not force them into existence.

That's yoga.
It's chai, not try.

Humor Break: Signs You're Trying Too Hard in Yoga

- You're holding your breath so fiercely during a pose, the teacher mistakes you for doing intense internal cleansing.

- You glance around mid-practice to compare your Down Dog to everyone else's, including the woman who looks like a retired ballerina fused with a rubber band.

- Your jaw is tighter than your hamstrings.

- You hear "Let go" and your brain goes, "Absolutely not. We have a schedule."

But Seriously, Why Is "Effortlessness" So Hard?

Blame evolution.
Our brains are wired for doing, not being.
Saber-toothed tigers didn't care about your mindfulness practice.
So trying — pushing, fixing, optimizing — is our default mode.

Effortlessness feels... suspicious.
Lazy.
Like if we're not gripping every muscle, life will fall apart.

But here's the paradox yoga reveals:
Sometimes, letting go IS the work.
Not collapsing. Not quitting. But *releasing the unnecessary.*

It's like cleaning out your junk drawer.
Do you need seven dried pens and a single chopstick? No.
Same goes for your habit of clenching your butt through Warrior II.

The Magic of Almost-Not-Trying

There's a moment — maybe in Savasana, maybe during a particularly juicy
twist — when you stop fighting the pose and it *just happens.*
Your breath deepens.
Your forehead un-frowns.
You're not pushing or striving. You're just... *there.*

And in that moment, you realize:
Trying was the thing that kept getting in the way.

Campfire Takeaway: Stir Gently

Life isn't a HIIT class. It's a slow-brewed cup of something sacred.

Yes, effort is part of yoga — tapas (discipline), after all, is real.
But so is ease. So is trust. So is making your movements feel like a
conversation instead of a debate.

So next time you're in a pose — or life throws you one — remember the
Chai Principle.

Simmer. Breathe. Let go of overdoing.
And if anyone asks what you're working on?

Tell them, proudly:

"Not trying too hard."

Then sip something warm and enjoy the silence like the enlightened little
gremlin you are.

Chapter 3: Krishnamacharya and the Breath That Launched a Thousand Flows

In which a quiet South Indian scholar changes the future of yoga, and we all learn that transitions are just as holy as destinations.

If yoga had a cinematic universe (and let's be honest, it probably should), Sri Tirumalai Krishnamacharya would be that wise, mysterious mentor figure — the Dumbledore, the Obi-Wan, the Gandalf — quietly responsible for nearly *everything* we associate with modern yoga.

He's the reason your Vinyasa class flows.
The reason your poses breathe.
The reason there's *any* structure behind your limbs flailing in what occasionally resembles grace.

But here's the twist: despite being the philosophical grandfather of Vinyasa, Krishnamacharya didn't set out to make yoga cool, commercial, or coordinated with Spotify playlists. He was a Sanskrit scholar, a healer, and a deeply traditional teacher whose real genius lay in his ability to merge the old with the new — to take the ancient wisdom of the yogic texts and make them move, literally, for modern bodies and modern minds.

And oh boy, did he move them.

First, Who Was This Guy?

Born in 1888 in South India, Krishnamacharya grew up devouring scriptures the way some kids devour cereal — joyfully, obsessively, and probably with better posture. By his twenties, he had mastered several of the key yogic texts, earned degrees in logic, Sanskrit, and Ayurveda, and had traveled to remote Himalayan caves to study with gurus who probably didn't even own shoes.

He was the full package:

> Scholar
> Practitioner
> Teacher
> Experimentalist
> Mystic
> And, according to some accounts, kind of a badass (he could stop his heartbeat on command).

Krishnamacharya wasn't interested in surface-level instruction. His yoga wasn't about trendy leggings or whether your Downward Dog looked cute on Instagram. It was about transformation — using breath, movement, discipline, and philosophy to fundamentally shift your experience of self and the world.

The Breath That Changed Everything

If Krishnamacharya had a catchphrase, it wouldn't be "Feel the burn" or "Engage your core." It would be something like:

"The breath is the boss."

Seriously, if yoga poses were musicians, the breath would be the conductor — guiding, shaping, and uniting the whole symphony. And Krishnamacharya knew this long before it became a buzzword in yoga teacher trainings.

In his system, no movement happened without breath.

- Inhale = expansion, lift, reach.

- Exhale = grounding, folding, surrender.
  Every pose, every transition, was woven with breath like a thread holding the whole tapestry together.

It wasn't about performing the fanciest poses — it was about moving intelligently, gradually, and with deep inner awareness, breath by breath.

Enter: Vinyasa Krama (a.k.a. "Yoga that Actually Makes Sense")

One of Krishnamacharya's greatest gifts to the yoga world was his concept of Vinyasa Krama. We touched on it earlier (you remember — the lasagna-sequencing metaphor), but now we get the full dish.

Krama means "steps" or "progression."
Vinyasa Krama = placing things (poses, breath, focus) in a thoughtful, sequential way.

Sounds obvious, right?

But before Krishnamacharya, a lot of yoga was either seated, still, or practiced as isolated poses with long holds. The idea of using movement as a progressive pathway — preparing the body systematically, transitioning with intention, and adapting the flow for individual needs — was revolutionary.

Think of it like building a playlist.
You don't start with the power ballad and then drop a lullaby.
You build. You rise. You release.
You flow.

That's Vinyasa Krama.

Movement Between Poses: The Lost Art We Owe to Krishnamacharya

Here's a fun fact that should be shouted from every yoga mat:

Krishnamacharya taught that the movement between the poses is as important as the pose itself.

Let that sink in.

So often we treat transitions like the "elevator music" of class — something to get through quickly so we can land in our next glorious Instagram-worthy pose. But to Krishnamacharya, *how* you got there was just as revealing, just as transformational, as the destination.

That little half-second when you float from plank to cobra?
Sacred.

That moment when you fall out of a balance pose, giggle, and reset?
Sacred.

That breath you take before folding forward?
Yep — still sacred.

Teacher of Teachers: His Legendary Students

Krishnamacharya's teachings birthed multiple yoga empires. His students — each brilliant in their own right — took pieces of his wisdom and spread them across the globe:

Pattabhi Jois

Took the flowing style and structured it into the Ashtanga system — fixed series, high discipline, and *lots* of jumping.

B.K.S. Iyengar

Focused on alignment, props, and precision. Turned yoga into a kind of anatomical poetry.

T.K.V. Desikachar

Krishnamacharya's son. Emphasized therapy, personalization, and breath-led sequencing. Called his approach Viniyoga, meaning "appropriate application."

Each one adapted Krishnamacharya's work in a different direction, like jazz musicians riffing on the same melody. That melody? The breath-led, step-by-step progression of Vinyasa.

Humor Break: If Krishnamacharya Taught a Modern Class

Imagine walking into your local studio, and there's an elderly Indian man sitting cross-legged with the stern patience of someone who's memorized the Vedas *and* survived raising teenagers.

He looks at your neon yoga mat.
Your stainless steel water bottle.
Your Bluetooth earbuds.

He smiles politely and says:

"We begin with the breath. And yes, I see your phone vibrating. Ignore it. Unless it's Brahman calling."

Campfire Takeaway: Transitions Are Sacred (Also, Mustaches Can Be Revolutionary)

Krishnamacharya didn't invent yoga.
He translated it for a new era.

He brought the ancient into the modern, the internal into the external, and most importantly, the breath into everything.

Without him, your Vinyasa class wouldn't flow. It would probably still be a series of static postures done in woolen robes by candlelight. (Which honestly sounds kinda cool but also kind of flammable.)

Because of him, yoga became living, adaptive, breath-centered movement — and every time you link a pose to your breath, you're participating in his legacy.

So next time you're in class, transitioning mindfully from Downward Dog to Lunge, or from chaos to calm, remember:

You are not just moving.
You are placing yourself — breath, body, and mind — in a special way.
You are walking in the footsteps of a scholar, healer, and teacher who knew that how we move through life is just as important as where we end up.

Chapter 4: Ashtanga, Flow, and Freestyle — Yoga's Greatest Remix Album

In which structure meets spontaneity, and we discover that all Vinyasa is family, even if some cousins are more intense than others.

There's a moment in every yogi's journey where you ask yourself:

"Wait, what kind of yoga *is* this?"

You look up from your mat, sweat dripping into your eye, trying to decipher if this is Vinyasa, Ashtanga, Power, Flow, Slow Flow, Vinyasa Fusion, or someone's creative expression of interpretive dolphin yoga.

Welcome to the modern yoga studio — part temple, part jungle gym, part spiritual identity crisis.

But here's the good news: they all share DNA. And that DNA traces back to one mustachioed man (you met him last chapter — Krishnamacharya), whose teachings gave rise to several wildly popular yoga styles.

What happened next was the yoga version of a family reunion where everyone brought their own casserole and insisted theirs was the original recipe. Spoiler: all delicious, all slightly different.

Let's Meet the Remix Artists

Krishnamacharya's three most famous students each took his teachings and ran with them — in different directions, tempos, and vibes. Let's break it down like your cool music-loving friend explaining the difference between jazz, funk, and lo-fi beats.

Ashtanga Vinyasa Yoga — The Discipline DJ

Student: Pattabhi Jois

If Vinyasa yoga were a playlist, Ashtanga would be that meticulously organized vinyl collection. No shuffling. No skipping. You do the full album, start to finish — and yes, that includes the weird track in the middle that no one likes but is somehow important for "growth."

Key Features:

- Set sequences (Primary, Intermediate, Advanced).

- Breath-synchronized movement (*vinyasa* between poses).

- Focus on Tristhana: breath (Ujjayi), gaze (Drishti), and energy locks (Bandhas).

- Lots of jumping. A bit of sweating. Occasional weeping.

Personality:
The Type-A yogi. Shows up early. Folds their yoga towel with military precision. Thinks a handstand is a reasonable way to start the day.

Why It Matters:
Ashtanga Vinyasa formalized the link between breath and movement into a system so structured it practically has a GPS. Almost every modern Vinyasa style owes its flowing nature to this practice — even the ones that swapped Sanskrit for Sia.

Iyengar Yoga — The Anatomical Architect

Student: B.K.S. Iyengar

If Ashtanga is a playlist, Iyengar Yoga is the acoustic unplugged version — slowed down, stripped of flash, and obsessively tuned.

Key Features:

- Static postures held for long durations.

- Precision in alignment. You *will* learn what your kneecap is doing.

- Props galore — blocks, straps, bolsters, and possibly a small armory of yoga furniture.

Personality:

The engineer yogi. Loves blueprints. Can tell you the angle of your femur in Triangle Pose. Is suspicious of "flow" unless every joint has been thoroughly briefed.

Why It Matters:

Iyengar may not *look* like Vinyasa, but it contributed profoundly to how we understand body mechanics in flow-based yoga. Every time your teacher says, "Knee over ankle," thank B.K.S.

Viniyoga — The Therapist in the Corner with a Cup of Tea

Student: T.K.V. Desikachar (Krishnamacharya's son)

Now we arrive at Viniyoga — not a brand, not a studio chain, but a methodology. It's the quiet cousin in the family who listens deeply and adjusts everything to suit your mood, your history, and your cranky lower back.

Key Features:

- Individualized practices.

- Emphasis on breath-first movement.

- Often includes chanting, meditation, and philosophical teachings.

- Therapy-focused. Yoga for the *whole* you, not just your hamstrings.

Personality:

The wise auntie who brings soup and asks how your *heart* is doing. Believes yoga should fit you, not the other way around.

Why It Matters:

Viniyoga reminds us that Vinyasa is not about keeping up — it's about tuning in. It's not about the pose, but the process. Desikachar brought compassion into sequencing, which modern Flow yoga carries forward — ideally with fewer ego pushups.

Enter: Flow Yoga — The Freestyle Rebel with a Spotify Account

Now we get to the offspring of the great remix: Modern Vinyasa Flow.

Inspired by Ashtanga's movement, Iyengar's intelligence, and Viniyoga's adaptability, Flow yoga emerged in the West like a breathy phoenix — equal parts discipline and dance, structure and creativity.

Key Traits:

- Unfixed sequences. Classes are designed by the teacher, often themed.

- Breath-movement synchronization remains central.

- Playlists. Creative transitions. Occasional interpretive flourishes.

Flow is what happens when:

- Ashtanga said: "Repeat this exact sequence forever."

- Iyengar said: "But make it anatomically precise."

- Desikachar said: "Make sure it suits the student."

- Flow said: "Cool. I'm going to put that in a blender, add music, and teach on rooftops at sunset."

And we love it for that.

"But Isn't That Watering Down the Tradition?"

Ah yes — the inevitable question. Is modern Flow yoga a betrayal of the past?

Here's the thing: *Tradition is not repetition. It's preservation through adaptation.* Krishnamacharya himself never taught the same class to two people. He adjusted based on constitution, season, mental state, and physical ability.

So when your local Vinyasa class includes cat-cow, an EDM remix of a mantra, and a heart-opening sequence that ends in laughter — that's not disrespect. That's evolution, baby.

It's tradition *alive*.

Humor Break: Yoga Styles as Family Members at a Reunion

- **Ashtanga**: Shows up with a spreadsheet. Finishes Savasana standing up.

- **Iyengar**: Brings their own folding chair. Corrects your posture at dinner.

- **Viniyoga**: Asks how your soul is doing. Actually listens.

- **Flow Yoga**: Arrives late but glowing. Brought a playlist and artisanal kombucha. Doesn't follow recipes but somehow nails the meal.

Campfire Takeaway: It's All One Song

Every yoga style you've tried — every teacher you've loved or side-eyed — is singing a different verse of the same song. That song is:

Breathe. Move. Notice. Connect.

Ashtanga gave us rhythm.
Iyengar gave us form.

Desikachar gave us soul.

Modern Flow gave us permission to remix it all.

So whether your practice is structured or spontaneous, sweaty or slow, silent or soundtracked — if you're linking breath with intention, you're in the family.

You're dancing in the long, beautiful lineage of Vinyasa.

And like any good remix, it's never about copying the original.
It's about honoring its heart while making it your own.

Interlude: Down Dog Diaries — Confessions from a Wobbly Warrior

In which we embrace the awkward, celebrate the shaky, and declare war on the myth of the Perfect Yogi.

Dear yoga journal,

It happened again.
I tried to flow gracefully from Warrior II to Half Moon Pose, but instead I looked like a drunk flamingo falling off a bar stool.

There was arm flailing. There was panic breathing. There was a moment where I might have made eye contact with my own foot.

And here's the kicker: no one cared.
Not even the teacher, who was too busy adjusting Chad's overzealous Wheel Pose in the back.

Myth: Yoga Makes You Graceful

Truth: Yoga Makes You Aware (Of How Uncoordinated You Are)

Let's be honest. Most of us didn't come to yoga for spiritual enlightenment. We came for:

- Back pain

- Stress relief

- The cute person from accounting who invited us

- Revenge on our tight hamstrings

- All of the above

And somewhere along the way, we were promised that we'd become serene, bendy, lotus-sitting beings who breathe evenly under pressure and own more linen than anxiety.

But here's the actual yoga journey:

1. Attend class.

2. Breathe deeply.

3. Sweat awkwardly.

4. Attempt a bind that turns you into a pretzel with self-doubt.

5. Accept your humanity.

6. Repeat.

Top 5 Awkward Yoga Moments (We've All Been There)

1. Falling out of Tree Pose… into your neighbor.

2. Doing Cat-Cow in the wrong direction. (You moo'd when everyone else meowed.)

3. Forgetting which leg goes forward. (And then pretending it was "intentional creative sequencing.")

4. Letting out a very questionable "breath" in Happy Baby.

5. Peeking during Savasana to see if others are "still relaxing correctly."

Let's Get Real: Nobody's Floating

Social media would have you believe that real yogis hover gracefully in handstands over cliff edges, sipping green juice with their chakras aligned like IKEA shelves.

But real yoga is messy.
It's the guy next to you who keeps sighing dramatically.
It's the teacher's mic dying mid-Sun Salutation.
It's realizing halfway through class that your leggings are on backwards —
and deciding to own it.

It's not about looking the part.
It's about showing up, even when you're wobbly, tired, or just deeply
confused about where your left foot went.

Humor Break: Yoga Class Archetypes

- The Heavy Breather: Sounds like Darth Vader in a wind tunnel.

- The Quiet Overachiever: Casually floats into Crow Pose while you
  struggle with child's pose and resentment.

- The Yogapologist: Constantly whispers "sorry" when adjusting their
  mat, sneezing, or existing.

- The Spiritual Literalist: Whispers "Namaste" before and after
  everything, including restroom breaks.

- You: Doing your best, breathing (mostly), and trying not to knock
  over the incense.

The Magic of Embracing the Wobble

The real heart of yoga isn't about being perfect — it's about being present.
And being present sometimes means being awkward, unsure, and giggling
mid-pose because your thigh just made a sound you didn't think was
physically possible.

Every time you wobble in Warrior III and don't give up — that's yoga.
Every time you fall out of Crow Pose and try again — that's yoga.

Every time you breathe through discomfort instead of bailing — that's yoga.

Campfire Takeaway: The Practice *Is* the Point

There's no final level.
No cosmic certificate of "You Did It, Yogi."
There's just the mat, the breath, the moment, and your weird, wonderful, imperfect body doing its very best.

So next time you topple out of a pose, grin.
Bow to the chaos.
And remember: every master was once a beginner who wobbled, too.

Especially in Downward Dog.

Chapter 5: The Holy Trifecta — Breath, Bandhas, and Drishti Walk Into a Bar

In which the core tools of Vinyasa get personified, spiritualized, and occasionally mocked with affection.

Imagine this:

You're in a dimly lit yoga bar (yes, we're going there), sipping something herbal and suspiciously murky. The door swings open. Three strangers walk in:

1. **Ujjayi Breath** — calm, oceanic, smells faintly of eucalyptus.

2. **Mula Bandha** — quiet, grounded, probably wearing all black and keeping an eye on everyone.

3. **Drishti** — laser focus, intense eye contact, doesn't blink.

They sit at the bar. The bartender raises an eyebrow and asks:

"What'll it be?"

Ujjayi sighs.

"Stillness, on the rocks."

Bandha murmurs:

"Control, neat."

Drishti locks eyes with the bartender and says:

"Awareness. Straight up."

The bartender, clearly rattled, just nods and pours them all a double shot of Vinyasa Enlightenment.

Welcome to the Tristhana method — the holy trifecta of breath, bandhas, and gaze.

These three elements are like the secret ingredients of Vinyasa. Not the Instagram-visible ones (like arm balances and very serene ponytails), but the deep, internal ones that turn your practice from a workout into a moving meditation.

They're what make Vinyasa more than just fancy stretching.
They're your anchors, your engine, and your internal GPS.
And together, they teach you how to be — right here, right now, in the middle of the movement.

The Breath (Ujjayi): Your Internal Metronome

Let's start with the breath — specifically, Ujjayi Pranayama, a.k.a. the "victorious breath."

What It Sounds Like:
The ocean in your throat.
Or Darth Vader with a PhD in mindfulness.

How You Do It:

- Slightly constrict the back of your throat (the glottis), as if whispering "haaaa" with your mouth closed.

- Inhale and exhale *through the nose* — slow, steady, slightly audible.

- Imagine your breath is both your soundtrack and your steering wheel.

Why It Matters:

Breath is *everything* in Vinyasa. Without it, you're just flailing with good intentions.

- It links movement to awareness.

- It activates your parasympathetic nervous system (that's the "rest and digest" one, not the "fight or flee because your phone buzzed" one).

- It generates internal heat — a.k.a. tapas — which isn't just good for a sweaty T-shirt pic; it's the fire of transformation.

And let's not forget:

Ujjayi is your anchor when things get spicy — on or off the mat.
Boss emails you 3 minutes before closing? Ujjayi.
Kid drops spaghetti on the dog? Ujjayi.
Holding Warrior II for the seventh breath and questioning your life choices? You know what to do.

The Bandhas: Internal Locks (a.k.a. The Unsung Heroes of Core Stability)

Next up: Bandhas — Sanskrit for "locks," or as I like to call them: *the inner bouncers of your energy nightclub.*

These subtle, muscular engagements help direct energy inward and upward, stabilize your body, and give your floating transitions that light, ninja-like feel — instead of the *thud-of-doom* we all know too well.

1. Mula Bandha — The Root Lock

Location: Pelvic floor

How to Engage It: Gentle lift of the perineum (like a Kegel with spiritual aspirations).

Why It's Important:

- Grounds you in balance poses.

- Supports your spine.

- Keeps energy from leaking out the basement floor of your being.

Fun Fact:

Mula Bandha is like your low-key best friend — doesn't talk much, but keeps you from collapsing at parties (or in Tree Pose).

2. Uddiyana Bandha — The Abdominal Lift

Location: Below the navel

How to Engage It: Draw the lower belly inward and slightly upward.

Why It's Important:

- Protects your lower back.

- Lifts your energy (and occasionally your butt) in jump-backs.

- Helps control transitions with ninja precision.

Reminder:

This is not a suck-in-your-gut "beach body" thing.
It's more like… hugging your organs with intention. (Trust me, it's classier than it sounds.)

3. Jalandhara Bandha — The Throat Lock

Location: Base of the throat

How to Engage It: Slight chin tuck — like you're nodding "hmm" at a philosophical podcast.

When You Use It: Mostly in seated breathing or pranayama practices, but it makes cameos in poses like Shoulderstand.

Why It Matters:

- Balances blood flow to the brain.

- Seals off upward movement of prana to keep energy circulating inward.

- Makes you look mildly mysterious in photos.

Drishti: The Power of a Gaze That Doesn't Wander

Finally, we meet Drishti — your focused gaze point.

Yes, it seems small. Yes, it can feel a bit intense.
But trust me, where you look affects where your mind goes.

Think of Drishti as:

- Your visual anchor.

- A flashlight for your awareness.

- A polite way to avoid checking out your neighbor's leggings mid-class.

In Ashtanga, there are nine official Drishtis (including your thumb, nose, and third eye), but the main goal is always the same: internal focus.

When your gaze settles, your monkey mind starts to chill.
You're no longer watching. You're witnessing.

Humor Break: How the Trifecta Shows Up in Real Life

- **Ujjayi:** You breathing deeply in traffic to avoid screaming at a red light.

- **Mula Bandha:** You clenching the pelvic floor as you try to hold in your opinion at Thanksgiving dinner.

- **Drishti:** You staring at a muffin during a work meeting, trying to practice detachment but failing gloriously.

Why These Three Matter (Like, Really Matter)

When used together, these three elements form the spiritual scaffolding of your practice.

- Ujjayi keeps you *present*.

- Bandhas keep you *contained*.

- Drishti keeps you *focused*.

They're not flashy.
They won't get you more likes.
But they will turn your practice into a living, breathing meditation — one where every inhale is sacred, every exhale a surrender, and every gaze a moment of mindfulness.

42

Campfire Takeaway: The Real Tools Are Internal

Let the CrossFit crowd keep their kettlebells.
Let the weekend warriors keep their Fitbits.

You? You've got the Tristhana Method.

You've got:

- A breath that sounds like waves and calms like therapy.

- An inner core that whispers "you're safe" even when your legs are trembling.

- A gaze that anchors you in the here and now, instead of the what-ifs and should-haves.

So the next time your teacher says, "Come back to your breath," or "Engage your bandhas," or "Fix your drishti," don't roll your eyes.

These aren't just technical cues.
They're invitations to presence.

And when you accept that invitation — breath by breath, bandha by bandha, blink by blink — something extraordinary happens:

You stop doing yoga… and start being yoga.

44

Chapter 6: Heat, Sweat, and Tapas — The Yoga of Mildly Controlled Suffering

In which we discover that sometimes burning from the inside out is exactly what the soul ordered.

There's a moment in most Vinyasa classes — usually about 20 minutes in, during your third chaturanga and second spiritual reckoning — when your body whispers, "Hey... what if we just *stop?*"

And your brain, ever the overachiever, replies:

"We can't. This is for *growth.*"

Then the teacher says, in their most serene voice:

"Stay with the discomfort. This is tapas."

And you, dripping, trembling, mildly hallucinating, think:

"I came here to feel *peace*, not *pain*, Sharon."

But here's the twist: tapas isn't punishment. It's purification.

It's the alchemical fire that burns away what you don't need, to reveal the part of you that's already whole.

It's yoga's spicy middle child — not as flashy as poses, not as cerebral as philosophy, but absolutely essential if you want your practice to do more than just tone your glutes.

Wait... Tapas? Like the Appetizers?

Nope. Sorry. Wrong spiritual buffet.

In yoga, tapas comes from the Sanskrit root *"tap"* — meaning to heat, to shine, to burn.

It refers to the inner fire of discipline, the intentional friction that awakens your awareness and melts away the sludge — mental, emotional, energetic, and sometimes literal (lookin' at you, hip tension from 2014).

Think of it like spiritual composting:

You take discomfort, resistance, ego, and a sprinkle of tight hamstrings, and let the heat of practice break them down into… clarity, strength, and calm.

Magic? No.

Science, discipline, and sweat? Absolutely.

Where Tapas Shows Up on the Mat

Contrary to popular belief, tapas isn't just holding plank until your soul leaves your body. It shows up subtly and powerfully across your entire practice:

1. Staying in the Pose When You Want to Flee

That moment in Warrior II when your thigh is screaming louder than your inner peace?
Tapas.

2. Returning to the Breath When Your Mind Is Planning Dinner

You want to mentally check out. But you don't. You *stay*.
Tapas.

3. Practicing Even When You're Not "Feeling It"

That Tuesday morning when you'd rather roll into a croissant than a cobra pose — but you still show up?
Yup. That's tapas too.

The Neuroscience of Heat and Habit

Science alert — don't worry, there's a metaphor coming.

When we engage in focused, challenging activities with deliberate discomfort, the brain lights up in fascinating ways.

- Neuroplasticity increases: You're literally rewiring your mind.

- Stress resilience improves: You're practicing emotional regulation.

- Dopamine becomes more balanced: Instead of constant craving, you find calm in the challenge.

In short, your brain learns:

"Oh, we can survive this. Maybe even grow from this."

Think of Tapas like Mental Strength Training:

- Tapas is the weight.

- Your mind is the muscle.

- Every breath you take instead of quitting = a rep.

And unlike that overpriced gym membership, yoga doesn't judge your outfit.

Humor Break: Top Signs You're Experiencing Tapas (and Not Just Low Blood Sugar)

- You start bargaining with your teacher telepathically. ("If I hold this pose, please skip the next vinyasa.")

- Your sweat forms its own lake system.

- You briefly reconsider all your life choices, especially the ones involving power yoga.

- You become spiritually bonded with the person next to you — not from eye contact, but shared suffering in Chair Pose.

- You leave class high on breath, sore in body, and suspiciously close to enlightenment.

Tapas Off the Mat: Life's Other Sweaty Lessons

Here's where yoga gets sneaky:
Tapas isn't just for the mat. It's how we grow *everywhere*.

- Showing up for hard conversations instead of ghosting?
Tapas.

- Holding your tongue when you want to "win" the argument?
Tapas.

- Saying no to something shiny so you can say yes to what matters?
Tapas.

It's not about suffering for suffering's sake.
It's about staying present in discomfort long enough to let it teach you something.

Fire As a Force of Clarity

In yogic mythology, fire is transformational. It's not destruction — it's refinement.

Agni, the fire god, doesn't burn you down.
He burns away what's not *you*.

Tapas is that same fire.
It clears out the noise.
It sharpens the soul.
It says, "Let's melt away the junk so the real you can shine."

48

And in a world full of shortcuts and dopamine hits, there's something radical about doing something *hard* on purpose — with kindness, not cruelty. With breath, not brute force.

A Note on Kindness (Because This Isn't a Bootcamp)

Let's be real: Some people hear "discipline" and go full Navy SEAL. Yoga says... maybe chill.

Tapas isn't punishment.
It's presence.
It's commitment.
It's choosing what serves your growth, even when it's not convenient or cute.

So no, you don't have to turn your mat into a battlefield.
But you do have to show up.
And keep showing up.
Even — especially — when it's hard.

Campfire Takeaway: Let Yourself Burn (A Little)

The goal of yoga isn't to become fireproof.
It's to become *fire-fed* — to let that internal heat clarify, cleanse, and connect you to something deeper than comfort.

Tapas is the quiet voice that says:

"You're strong enough to stay."
"You're awake enough to grow."
"You're brave enough to feel this."

And as you move, sweat, breathe, and occasionally collapse into Child's Pose whispering "why," just remember:

You're not falling apart.
You're burning away what no longer serves.

One chaturanga at a time.

Chapter 7: Vinyasa Krama — Building a Sequence Like Grandma Builds a Lasagna

In which we discover that yoga sequencing is less like a workout plan and more like Italian cooking with cosmic undertones.

First, What *Is* Vinyasa Krama?

Let's break this down like noodles on a countertop.

- Vinyasa = to place in a special way (remember our sandwich metaphor? Still relevant.)

- Krama = step-by-step progression.

Put it together and you get:

"To place things in a special way, step by step."

In other words: Don't just fling your poses around like a yoga salad. Build them like layers of meaning — one careful step at a time.

And yes, I'm going to keep comparing it to lasagna. You've been warned.

The Problem With "Random Yoga"

Let's be real. We've all been in That Class™:

You start in Child's Pose, suddenly you're in a handstand, and then boom — seated forward fold. Somewhere in there was a Warrior 3 that required a level of hamstring forgiveness you just didn't have that day.

It's like a yoga smoothie — well-intentioned, but possibly confusing and full of ingredients that don't belong together.

Krishnamacharya — our wise, breath-obsessed, sequencing-obsessed grandmaster — believed this was yoga blasphemy.

To him, every practice needed a trajectory. A clear journey. A beginning, middle, and end. Like a meal. Or a novel. Or yes, a *well-layered, bubbling lasagna of transformation.*

Grandma's Lasagna and Krishnamacharya's Yoga: A Comparative Guide

Grandma's Lasagna	Vinyasa Krama
Sauce first — always lay the base.	Start with grounding — breath, intention, gentle flow.
Then noodles — structure begins.	Add in foundational poses: Sun Salutations, standing.
Cheese, sauce, repeat.	Build complexity — backbends, balances, deeper work.
Top with care — nothing random.	Finish with cool-downs, forward folds, hip openers.
Bake — give it time.	Savasana — let it settle, let it integrate.
Serve with love.	Close with breath, reflection, gratitude.

How a Thoughtful Sequence Works

Let's look under the lid of this metaphorical casserole dish and explore common sequencing strategies in Vinyasa Krama:

1. The Peak Pose Model

Build toward one juicy, challenging pose (like a King Pigeon or Flying Something-or-Other).

Why it works:

- Every pose before it prepares the body.
- It's satisfying AF to finally arrive.
- You don't die in the process (ideally).

Lasagna Equivalent:

You don't put ricotta on raw noodles and hope for the best. You prep, layer, and build to gooey perfection.

2. Anatomical Focus

Today's class is all about hips, or spine mobility, or core strength (a.k.a. your least favorite part).

Why it works:

- Specific.
- Intentional.
- Less likely to accidentally overstretch something important.

Lasagna Equivalent:

Know what kind of cheese you're using. Don't toss in marshmallows and call it "creative."

---

3. Energetic or Philosophical Themes

Your sequence matches a *state* of being: grounding, opening, letting go, joy, fire, water, air, Beyoncé energy.

Why it works:

- Adds depth.

- Connects physical to emotional/spiritual.

- Students leave feeling seen, not just stretched.

Lasagna Equivalent:

The secret ingredient is always love. Or wine. But mostly love.

Why This All Matters (Beyond Being Delicious)

Your nervous system *craves sequence*. It wants to feel:

- Safe → So you start slow.

- Challenged → So you build smart.

- Integrated → So you end soft.

A random sequence might still be *hard* — but it's not harmonized.

Vinyasa Krama is like being handed a roadmap instead of wandering around the yoga wilderness hoping you don't sprain your third eye.

Humor Break: Signs a Class Lacks Krama

- You go from Savasana to Crow Pose in three breaths.

- The teacher's cue is "Do whatever feels right" and you're like, "Well, leaving seems right."

- You realize halfway through that the class is just a string of your teacher's favorite poses (including three Camels and zero warm-ups).

- You spend 15 minutes on wrist-heavy poses with *no* wrist prep and start fantasizing about suing them in Small Claims Chakra Court.

The Deeper Layer: Krama as a Life Philosophy

This isn't just about yoga. It's about how you do anything.

- You don't build a relationship by jumping to deep vulnerability on day one.

- You don't start your career with a TED Talk (unless you're a very precocious child).

- You don't find peace by forcing yourself to be peaceful.

Krama says: One step. Then another. Each one placed in a special way.

Vinyasa Krama in Everyday Life (a.k.a. The Lasagna of Living)

- Morning routine → Start slow, add complexity. (Don't check emails before teeth-brushing. Come on.)

- Conflict → Breathe, ground, then speak.

- Healing → Don't rush. Layer gentleness with truth. Let it bake.

Campfire Takeaway: Don't Skip the Sauce

In a world of shortcuts and 30-minute express yoga, Vinyasa Krama invites you to slow down and build something with love.

Not because it's trendy.
Not because it makes you more "advanced."
But because it teaches you how to respect the process — on the mat and in your life.

So next time you're tempted to jump from Down Dog into something dramatic without preparation, pause.

Ask yourself:

"Have I sauced this sequence with care?"
"Have I layered in breath, focus, and foundation?"

If yes — welcome to the yoga kitchen, maestro.

Now take a deep breath…
And keep layering.

Chapter 8: Why Your Hamstrings Hate You (And What Patañjali Has to Say About It)

In which we unpack physical tension, emotional baggage, spiritual resistance, and what stretching has to do with surrender.

There you are, halfway into a seemingly innocent seated forward fold. Legs extended, toes flexed, spine reaching. Your teacher says, "Gently fold forward."

But your hamstrings — those sneaky ropes of rebellion — say,

"Gently? *Gently?!* We don't do gently. We do screaming."

You inch forward.

They inch backward.

Suddenly, your yoga mat becomes a battleground, your hamstrings the gatekeepers of some ancient, unresolved grievance you didn't know you were carrying until now.

And that, dear reader, is where the wisdom of Patañjali comes in.

Because as it turns out, *stretching isn't just about the body.*
It's about your relationship to resistance.
And no one explained that better than a bearded sage who never Instagrammed a single pose.

Meet Patañjali: The Godfather of Yogic Psychology

Patañjali — not to be confused with the budget Ayurvedic toothpaste brand — was the ancient compiler of the Yoga Sūtras, a collection of pithy, poetic, and sometimes maddeningly vague aphorisms that lay the psychological groundwork of yoga.

His thesis, if we may be so bold, can be summarized as:

"Your mind is messy. Still it."

Sutra 1.2 hits you right in the Vrittis (mental fluctuations):

Yogaś citta-vṛtti-nirodhaḥ

"Yoga is the cessation of the fluctuations of the mind."

In other words, the goal of yoga isn't to get your heels to the mat in Down Dog.

It's to quiet the storm between your ears — the stories, judgments, fears, to-do lists, inner critiques, and hamstring-related curses.

So… Where Do Hamstrings Fit Into That?

Glad you asked.

Let's return to that seated forward fold. You're there, feeling stiff and annoyed. Your ego is whispering,

"Look at that guy over there touching his forehead to his shins. He probably composts."

And that's the moment — not when you fold, not when you "achieve" the pose — but when you notice the thoughts — that yoga begins.

Your hamstrings are not the obstacle.
They're the mirror.

They reflect your:

- Impatience ("I should be deeper!")

- Ego ("I used to be more flexible before that one time I tried CrossFit.")

- Self-judgment ("Why am I like this?")

- Control issues ("If I just force it harder, it'll surrender!")

Which is exactly why they're so valuable.
Because you don't overcome resistance by defeating it.
You overcome it by meeting it.

That's yoga. And that's Patañjali's jam.

Humor Break: Things Your Hamstrings Would Say If They Could Talk

- "Oh you want to touch your toes? Cute."

- "We store your emotional baggage and we're unionized."

- "You sit for 9 hours a day and then expect us to open up like an Instagram influencer on day three of a silent retreat?"

- "We're not tight. You're just impatient."

Sutras That Secretly Explain Stretching Woes

Let's look at a few golden nuggets from Patañjali's Yoga Sūtras that make sense of your reluctant posterior chain.

1. Sutra 1.12 — Abhyāsa and Vairāgya

"Practice and non-attachment are the means to still the mind."

Translation for tight-hamstring moments:
Keep practicing.
Don't be attached to whether or not your nose touches your knees.
Every breath is the real win.

59

2. Sutra 2.46 — Sthira Sukham Āsanam

"The posture should be steady and comfortable."

Wait… comfortable?

Yes. Steady and comfortable. Not "pushed beyond all logic because your Type-A brain needs to win yoga."

This sutra is a reminder that asana isn't a performance — it's a relationship. One built on trust, not force.
You meet the edge, not bulldoze it.

3. Sutra 2.1 — Tapas, Svādhyāya, Īśvarapraṇidhāna

"Discipline, self-study, and surrender to the divine — these are yoga in practice."

Let's break this one down in forward fold terms:

- Tapas = You keep showing up, even when your hamstrings have a personal vendetta.

- Svādhyāya = You observe your thoughts in the pose instead of reacting to them.

- Īśvarapraṇidhāna = You surrender the outcome, trusting that the pose is enough, right now, as it is.

Sound familiar? Yep. It's the whole Vinyasa path — boiled down to one stiff-legged experience.

Why Flexibility Isn't the Goal (But Awareness Is)

In Western yoga culture, flexibility often becomes the unspoken measure of "success." We equate deep backbends and bendy splits with enlightenment, when in fact…

Flexibility is just a party trick. Presence is the point.

What good is touching your toes if you're thinking about emails while doing it?
What good is folding deeper if you're secretly hating yourself along the way?

Patañjali says:

It's not how far you go — it's how aware you are while you're there.

Hamstrings as the Portal to Humility

You know what hamstrings do really, really well?

They humble us.

They remind us that growth takes time. That surrender can be stronger than pushing. That a body isn't a machine — it's a storybook. And sometimes, a really tight one.

The tension you feel in your body is often just the echo of unexamined expectations. And yoga — good, honest, uncomfortable yoga — invites you to hear that echo, breathe with it, and let it soften.

Eventually.

No rush.

Campfire Takeaway: The Pose Is the Teacher, Not the Trophy

Your hamstrings might never love you. That's okay.

But if they help you:

- Slow down

- Let go

- Observe your mind

- Stay with discomfort

- Laugh at your impatience

…then they've already done their job.

So the next time you fold forward and feel that familiar resistance, smile.
You've met your teacher.
Now breathe, stay, and listen.

Patañjali would be proud.

Interlude: Yoga Class Is Weird and So Are We

A non-denominational tribute to everyone who's ever put their foot in the wrong place, their mat in the wrong spot, or their heart into a practice they don't fully understand.

Let's just say it out loud:
Yoga class is weird.

It's beautiful, transcendent, ancient, wise…
But also: deeply weird.

Where else in modern life are you expected to:

- Lie on the floor with strangers in the dark?

- Chant syllables you don't fully understand with a room full of sweaty accountants and baristas?

- Let someone gently press on your sacrum while you try not to fart?

No one tells you that yoga is 40% breath, 30% listening to your own stomach gurgle, 20% trying not to look at anyone's feet, and 10% quietly wondering if this is what cults feel like *but in a good way.*

Scene: You Walk Into a New Yoga Studio

You take your shoes off with nervous reverence — as if your footwear has committed sins.

You walk into the room like you're entering a library staffed by angels.

You place your mat with excessive precision, trying not to block anyone's sacred foot flow.

Someone's already warming up with a full headstand and what appears to be a breath of fire exorcism.

You, meanwhile, are wondering if you can still exit without drawing attention.

You sit.

You breathe.

And suddenly a soft voice says:

"Let your awareness melt into the back of your heart."

And you think:

"Um. Excuse me? Melt? *Into* it?? What even is the back of my heart?"

But you nod like you totally get it.
Because you're polite.
And also 12% afraid of the person next to you who appears to be levitating.

The Unspoken Yoga Class Archetypes

- The Groaner — Expresses every pose like it's a childbirth flashback.

- The Equipment Maximalist — Carries six blocks, two straps, a bolster, and a foam roller... for a 45-minute flow.

- The Sweater — Leaves a damp outline on their mat shaped like a confused bat.

- The Philosopher — Quotes Rumi after class and probably smells like patchouli and deep thoughts.

- You — Wondering if it's okay to ask what "chaturanga" means... during chaturanga.

Humor Break: Weird Things We All Pretend Are Normal in Yoga

- Being told to "shine your collarbones."

- Holding your big toe like it owes you money.

- The awkward moment of eye contact in Savasana (we weren't *supposed* to peek, but here we are).

- The studio playlist randomly dropping a didgeridoo solo over rain sounds and hip-hop.

- Clapping for the teacher at the end like they just won a Tony.

And yet…

We keep coming back.

Why?

Because Yoga Is Also Home for the Misfits

Yoga class is where:

- The overthinkers come to breathe.

- The stiff-backed desk warriors come to unfold.

- The anxious, the grieving, the joyful, the curious — all gather to be *a little more here* and *a little less tangled*.

Yes, it's weird.
But it's our kind of weird.
The kind that says, "You don't have to be perfect — just present."

The Unspoken Contract of the Mat

When you roll out your mat — whether it's pristine and Instagram-worthy or smells vaguely of dog — you're making a quiet agreement:

"I'll meet myself as I am today.
I won't win. I won't lose.
I'll wobble, sweat, laugh, fall, breathe... and maybe, just maybe, feel okay in my skin for a minute."

And everyone else in the room?
They're doing the same thing.

Probably also wondering if they locked their car.

Campfire Takeaway: Come As You Are (But Bring Snacks)

Yoga is ancient, sacred, powerful...
and also sometimes silly, uncomfortable, and confusing as hell.

That's okay.

The beauty is in the showing up.
The weirdness is part of the wisdom.
The awkwardness is just your soul stretching.

So roll out your mat.
Laugh when you fall.
Sigh when you land.
And remember:

You belong here. Even when you're facing the wrong direction.

Chapter 9: The Bhagavad Gita vs. Your Ego — The Pose Is Not the Point

In which we realize the mat is a battlefield, the war is mostly in our minds, and yoga isn't about winning... unless it's over yourself.

Scene One: A Warrior Has a Breakdown

Let's start with a story, one with less spandex and more chariots.

The Bhagavad Gita opens on a battlefield. Two massive armies are lined up for war. The air is thick with tension, dust, and questionable ethics. Arjuna, a skilled warrior, is in his chariot, bow in hand, muscles coiled. He looks across the battlefield and sees something truly horrifying:

His relatives.
His teachers.
People he loves.

And then?
He puts his weapons down and has an emotional breakdown. In full armor. On the battlefield.

Let that image sink in:
A literal warrior, crumbling under the weight of conflicted duty and paralyzing self-doubt.

Enter Krishna.
Arjuna's charioteer, spiritual counselor, and, plot twist — God in disguise.

Krishna doesn't say, "Get over it."
He says, "This war is inside you. Let's talk."

And that's how the Gita begins:

With existential dread in the middle of a to-do list.

Sound familiar?

Your Mat Is a Battlefield

Yoga is often sold as a peaceful, candlelit, lavender-scented oasis. And yes, it *can* be that.

But ask any long-term practitioner and they'll tell you:

The real yoga starts when things get messy.

When you're shaking in Warrior II and your brain says, "Why are we doing this again?"
When you try meditating and your mind turns into a Greatest Hits album of anxieties.
When you hold a pose longer than your ego thinks is reasonable, and your thoughts start yelling like toddlers denied a snack.

That, my friend, is your Arjuna moment.

The battlefield is your mat.
The opposing armies? Your ego and your essence.
And the Gita is here to tell you:

Stop aiming for the perfect pose. Start practicing skillful action without attachment to results.

The Gita's Main Mic Drop: Karma Yoga

In Chapter 2, Verse 47, Krishna delivers the quote that could be printed on every yoga mat:

"You have the right to the action, not to the fruits of the action."

Translation:

Do the work. Let go of the outcome.

So simple.
So impossible.
So… yoga.

What That Looks Like in Class:

- You show up.

- You do the pose.

- You fall out of the pose.

- You don't spiral into shame.

- You laugh. You breathe. You try again.

You let the pose be the vehicle, not the destination.

Humor Break: When Your Ego Teaches Yoga Class

- "You should be deeper in this stretch."

- "You used to be more flexible before that cheese phase."

- "Why is your Ujjayi breath wheezing like a haunted radiator?"

- "Don't let them see you rest. CHILD'S POSE IS DEFEAT."

- "Do another vinyasa, even though you're clearly dying. Prove you're spiritual!"

That voice? That's your internal Arjuna, mid-freak-out.

The Gita says:

"Yeah, we all have one. Now breathe through it and keep going."

Detachment: Not Indifference, But Inner Freedom

In yoga, detachment doesn't mean apathy.
It means you do the thing because it's right — not because it strokes your self-image.

You stretch not to impress, but to feel.
You flow not to conquer the sequence, but to participate in presence.
You meditate not to achieve enlightenment by Tuesday, but to see what's *already* there when the noise dies down.

This is Karma Yoga:

Skill in action, minus the emotional baggage.

Ego Isn't Evil. It's Just... Loud.

Let's give ego a little compassion.
It's not trying to ruin your yoga. It's trying to protect you — by clinging to control, certainty, and comfort.

But yoga says:

"Discomfort isn't failure. It's the edge of transformation."

In that moment when your thighs are shaking, your balance is wonky, and your inner critic is screaming, you have a choice:

- Collapse into the drama.

- Or stand in the fire and breathe anyway.

That's Arjuna's choice.
That's your choice, every class.

The Pose Is Not the Point

Read that again.

It's the intention inside the pose.
The breath inside the effort.
The clarity inside the chaos.

The Gita tells us:

"Don't perform yoga. Live it.
Practice for the sake of the practice.
Do what is yours to do — and release the rest."

Campfire Takeaway: Win the Inner Battle, Not the Outer Pose

Your yoga mat is a chariot.
Every class is a conversation.
And the real question isn't, "Did I nail the pose?"
It's, "Did I act with presence, integrity, and love — even when it was hard?"

That's what Arjuna learned.
That's what the Gita teaches.
That's what your ego resists — and your soul quietly longs for.

So pick up your metaphorical bow, roll out your mat, and step into the arena.

The only thing you're being asked to conquer... is you.

And that?
That's the kind of victory that matters.

Chapter 10: Hatha Yoga, Prana Plumbing, and the Energetic Body

In which we tour the subtle systems beneath the skin, learn why you might feel weepy in pigeon pose, and discover that energy doesn't care how tight your hamstrings are.

First Off: You Are Not Just a Sack of Muscles

If you've ever cried in hip openers or felt euphoric after Savasana, congratulations — you've had a sneak peek into the energetic body, that quiet little system no MRI can see but every mystic swears by.

In the world of Hatha Yoga — the older cousin of Vinyasa — your body isn't just flesh and bone.
It's a bio-psycho-spiritual highway, with:

- Nadis (energy channels)

- Prana (life force)

- Chakras (energy hubs)

- And the occasional existential traffic jam.

Think of it as plumbing meets spirituality — with less leaking, more glowing.

What Is Prana (and Can I Put It in My Smoothie)?

Prana is often translated as "life force" — the subtle energy that animates us. Not just breath, but the thing *behind* the breath. The animating *oomph* in your cells.

In Western lingo, it's kinda like:

- Qi (in Chinese medicine)

- Mana (in Polynesian culture)

73

- The Force (in *Star Wars*, obviously)

Without prana, you're just a well-organized meat puppet. With prana, you're a living, breathing, twitchy miracle.

Meet the Nadis: Your Inner Energy Wires

Nadis (from Sanskrit, meaning "flow" or "tube") are the subtle channels that prana moves through.

Ancient texts say there are 72,000 of them. Because of course there are. Yogis don't do minimalism.

But really, we focus on three big ones:

1. Ida Nadi — The Lunar Channel

- Left side
- Cooling, calming, introspective
- Feminine energy
- Think: Moonlight, chamomile tea, and quiet journaling with a cat

2. Pingala Nadi — The Solar Channel

- Right side
- Heating, energizing, action-oriented
- Masculine energy
- Think: Sunlight, espresso, conquering your inbox before 9am

3. Sushumna Nadi — The Central Channel

- Runs up the spine
- The spiritual fast lane

- Where the magic happens (a.k.a. awakening, insight, enlightenment, and occasional unexplainable tingling)

In a balanced state, prana flows freely.
When blocked?
Welcome to tension, fatigue, anxiety, and the irrational urge to cry during pigeon.

Humor Break: Signs Your Nadis Need a Tune-Up

- You get annoyed at someone chewing too loudly, but cry at yogurt commercials.

- Your mood swings faster than your Spotify playlist.

- You feel "off" but can't explain it — so you deep-clean your closet instead.

- You wake up exhausted, go to sleep wired, and meditate like a squirrel with a caffeine habit.

So Where Does Hatha Yoga Come In?

Hatha Yoga isn't just "yoga with poses" — it's a full-on energy management system.

"Ha" = Sun (Pingala)
"Tha" = Moon (Ida)

So Hatha Yoga is literally the union of opposites: heat and cool, effort and ease, espresso and naps.

The goal isn't just to get stronger or more flexible — it's to:

- Balance your energy.

- Clear the blockages.

- Prepare the subtle body for higher states of awareness.

And how do we do that?

Through… you guessed it:

Asana. Pranayama. Bandhas. Drishti.

(Yes, all the tools we've already lovingly roasted in earlier chapters.)

Poses as Plumbing Tools

Every posture in Vinyasa — from the most casual Cat-Cow to the spicy Revolved Triangle — is designed to open, release, and redirect prana.

Here's how it works (very scientifically-ish):

- Backbends = Stimulate energy, lift mood, bust through chest blocks

- Forward folds = Soothe the nervous system, release back-of-the-body tension

- Twists = Squeeze-and-release your organs like stress balls (you're welcome)

- Inversions = Flip the script, reboot your system, feel like a bat

The sequencing (remember our lasagna?) is about clearing pathways step by step — so that when you sit in meditation, your mind isn't a circus.

It's clean. Clear. Flowing.

Like prana after a psychic colonic.

Bandhas and Breath: The Surge Protectors

Remember the bandhas (those energy locks we met in Chapter 5)?

- They're like valves, directing the energy upward instead of letting it leak out through your feet, your thoughts, or your grocery list.

- Combine them with Ujjayi breath, and suddenly you're not just doing yoga — you're moving light through your body.

No pressure or anything.

Chakras: Bonus Round (A.K.A. the Yogic Energy Apps)

Let's not go full chakra-deep here (that's another book and probably a subscription plan), but know this:

- Your spine houses not just your discs, but your potential.

- The chakras are energy centers along that spine — seven major ones — each governing physical, emotional, and spiritual aspects.

- When prana flows freely through them, you feel clear, creative, grounded, and alive.

When they're blocked?
You feel... well... like a cranky hose.

Real Talk: Can I *Feel* Prana?

Yes.

It's the tingle in your palms after a long Down Dog.
It's the heat behind your eyes after a deep meditation.
It's the moment in Savasana when your body is still but you feel wildly alive.

You don't need to *believe* in prana.
You just need to notice.

(Like tofu, it takes on the flavor of your awareness.)

Campfire Takeaway: You're Wired for Wonder

Your body isn't just skin, bones, and complaints.

It's a multi-layered marvel — physical on the outside, electric on the inside, spiritual at the core.

Hatha and Vinyasa Yoga give you the tools to clear the clutter, charge the system, and restore the current.

- Poses move energy.

- Breath directs it.

- Stillness refines it.

And suddenly, you're not just doing yoga.
You're becoming a conduit for something much bigger than yourself.

Call it prana.
Call it life.
Call it "that thing I feel in pigeon pose that makes me cry and also want to text my ex."

Whatever it is —
It's flowing now.

Interlude: Who Stole My Yoga Sock? A Domestic Mystery in Three Acts

A thrilling tale of loss, suspicion, and inner peace betrayed by laundry.

Act I: The Disappearance

It begins like all great spiritual crises do — subtly.

One cold morning, you rise for practice, muscles stiff, heart open, soul yearning for nothing more than a warm toe cocoon. You reach into your yoga drawer — the one filled with your sacred leggings, your crumpled headbands, and your designated fancy yoga socks (the ones with the sticky dots on the soles and the faint smell of eucalyptus).

You pull one out.
And… that's it.

One. Sock.

The other has vanished.

Not rolled under the bed.
Not tangled in your towel.
Not stuffed in a sleeve by your chaotic-but-lovable cat.

Gone.
Like enlightenment during rush hour.

And suddenly, the room is not a sanctuary.
It is a crime scene.

Act II: The Investigation

Fueled by indignation and caffeine, you launch a full-scale investigation.

Suspect #1: The Laundry Machine
Always hungry. Always spinning. Possibly a portal to another dimension where yoga socks, missing pens, and your youthful optimism all reside.

You dig through the lint trap.
You interrogate your dryer with fierce side-eye.
You even stick your hand down that weird, rubbery gasket gap that feels like it was designed by a trickster god.

Nothing.

Suspect #2: Your Partner/Roommate/Pet

You approach them casually.

"Hey, have you seen my grippy yoga sock?"

They reply with the blank, innocent stare of the truly guilty.

You squint.
They squint.
The tension is palpable.

They deny everything.
You say, "It's fine," but your tone suggests it is absolutely not fine.

Act III: Acceptance (Sort Of)

Days pass.
You practice sockless.
Your left foot sticks.
Your right foot slides.
Your Sun Salutations become a physical metaphor for imbalance and mild rage.

Then, one evening, as you're folding laundry you don't even remember washing, you find it:

The sock.

Stuck inside a fitted sheet.
Like it had been hiding.
Like it wanted to be found — but only on its own mystical terms.

You hold it in your hand.
It smells faintly of lavender and betrayal.

You stare into the middle distance and whisper,

"I forgive you."

And just like that...
You are enlightened.

Humor Break: Other Mystical Yoga Mysteries Yet Unsolved

- Where does your water bottle go during Savasana?

- Why do yoga mats age in dog years?

- Who turned up the heat when it was already hot yoga?

- Why does one nostril always breathe better than the other?

- And seriously... where *do* all the eye pillows go?

Campfire Takeaway: It Was Never About the Sock

Okay, fine — it was *a little* about the sock.

But really, it's about how we handle life's tiny, ridiculous inconveniences:

- With curiosity instead of control.

- With breath instead of blame.

- With laughter instead of panic.

Because yoga isn't just practiced on a mat.
It's practiced in your laundry room, your living room, your living soul.

And every missing sock, missed pose, or moment of imbalance is just another chance to practice:

Presence.
Patience.
And letting go of what you *thought* needed to happen so you could notice what *is* happening.

So the next time something small derails your inner peace — the sock, the burnt toast, the parking spot stolen by a guy named Chad — pause.

Breathe.

Maybe laugh.

And know:
You're still doing yoga.
Even when you're just folding laundry and forgiving your dryer.

Chapter 11: Modern Yoga Soup — Flow, Power, Yin, and the Great Buffet of Bendy Beliefs

The Yoga Buffet Problem

Let's say you're standing in front of an all-you-can-eat buffet.

There's sushi. And lasagna. And a taco bar.

A lady next to you is building a "fusion wrap" with falafel, mac 'n cheese, and jalapeños. You're overwhelmed. Excited. Slightly afraid.

Now replace the food with yoga styles, and welcome to the 21st-century yoga world.

Because if you're practicing yoga in the modern West, you're not just doing "yoga" — you're navigating an ever-expanding buffet of bendy beliefs.

Power Yoga. Yin Yoga. Rocket Yoga. Broga. Hot Flow. Slow Flow. Yoga Sculpt. Laughter Yoga. Goat Yoga. (Yes, we will eventually address the goats.)

What's going on here?

What happened to just... yoga?

Flashback: When Yoga Wasn't a Smorgasbord

Once upon a time — and by that, I mean pre-1970s — yoga in the West meant something relatively simple. A quiet mat, maybe a candle, and a teacher who whispered Sanskrit in between telling you to "breathe through the discomfort."

You'd show up, do your sun salutations, lie in Savasana, and go home blissed-out with a new appreciation for your hamstrings.

Then came the wellness boom. The fitness craze. The rise of Instagram. And suddenly, yoga needed to be **marketable**.

"Stretch your body and burn calories while achieving inner peace, enlightenment, and sculpted abs — all in 60 minutes or less!"

The result? Yoga turned into **Soup of the Day** — something new each time, depending on who's stirring the pot.

Modern Styles on the Menu

Let's break down what's currently in your typical yoga buffet — from the deeply traditional to the deeply...well, creative.

Power Yoga

Developed in the U.S. by folks like Beryl Bender Birch and Bryan Kest, Power Yoga is Vinyasa Yoga's high-energy cousin. Think of it as **Ashtanga after three espressos**. You sweat, you flow, you maybe cry in a plank pose. It's fitness-forward, often breath-informed, but sometimes... breath-forgotten.

Yin Yoga

Slow, still, and soul-probing. Yin asks you to **sit with discomfort** — holding passive floor poses for 3–7 minutes. It's like being gently mugged by your own hip flexors. Based on Taoist philosophy and meridian theory, it focuses on fascia and internal energy. Yin's the style most likely to make you cry and say thank you.

Hot Yoga

You know this one. A heated room. Sweaty bodies. Slippery mats. Often associated with Bikram or Power Vinyasa, Hot Yoga is sometimes transformational... and sometimes just *moist suffering*. Not for the faint of hydration.

Restorative Yoga

The gentle giant of the yoga world. Think: blankets, bolsters, pillows — and the blissful sensation of doing almost nothing while someone tells you you're doing it perfectly. It's basically a spa day disguised as spirituality.

Yoga Sculpt

Yoga with weights. Because clearly chaturanga wasn't hard enough. A high-intensity fusion class for those who like their yoga with a side of squats and EDM.

Goat Yoga

It exists. That's all I'll say. If you like Downward Goat, be my guest.

Humor Break: Yoga Class Types as Food Orders

- **Power Yoga** = spicy ramen with extra sriracha.
- **Yin Yoga** = slow-cooked stew your grandma makes when you're sad.
- **Hot Yoga** = ghost pepper chili eaten in a sauna.
- **Restorative Yoga** = mashed potatoes, under a blanket, with a candle lit.
- **Yoga Sculpt** = kale smoothie, shot of espresso, and a motivational speech.
- **Goat Yoga** = trail mix, but it climbs on your back.

Why So Many Styles?

Short answer? Capitalism.

Longer answer? A combination of:

- **Cultural evolution**
- **Commercial pressure**
- **Social media**
- **Diverse student needs**
- **A genuine desire to modernize and make yoga accessible**

The buffet exists because yoga's been democratized — and monetized. Everyone wants a taste, and teachers want to feed that hunger. That's not necessarily bad. Choice is good. Innovation can be great.

But here's the issue:

When yoga becomes a menu of experiences without any philosophical spine, it loses its heart.

If the breath is an afterthought…
If presence is sacrificed for performance…
If it's just stretching and sweating to look good in leggings…

Then we've drifted away from the original dish.

What Makes It *Still* Yoga?

This is where Traditional Vinyasa saves the day like a wise elder with soup and stories.

Despite all the remixing, yoga remains yoga **if** it includes:

- **Intention** (Are you practicing with awareness or autopilot?)
- **Breath** (Are you syncing movement and mind?)
- **Self-Inquiry** (Are you more connected when you finish than when you began?)
- **Surrender** (Are you open to letting go of the outcome?)

You can have all the fusion, variety, and Beyoncé-backbend mashups you want — but if the practice still points inward, you're on the right mat.

How to Navigate the Buffet Without Bellyache

1. Know Your Why.

What's your goal? Movement? Healing? Peace?
Choose accordingly.

2. Try Everything Once. Maybe Twice.

A "meh" class today could be exactly what you need next week.

3. Beware the Style Wars.

Some purists will say only [insert lineage here] is "real yoga." Smile. Breathe. Flow on.

4. Stick With What Grounds You.

Find the style or teacher that brings you back to **yourself**, not your ego.

5. Laugh at It Sometimes.

Yes, there's sacredness in yoga. But also… have you ever seen a grown adult fall asleep snoring in child's pose? Humor belongs here too.

Campfire Takeaway

Modern yoga is a big pot of stew.

Sometimes it's soulful and spiced with ancient wisdom.
Sometimes it's trendy tofu topped with kale-dusted hashtags.
But you know what?

The core ingredient is YOU.

Your breath. Your body. Your intention. Your awareness.

No matter what style you try — from sacred Sanskrit chanting to squats with goats — if you return to stillness and presence, you're still practicing yoga.

So dig in. Sample the soup.
But don't forget the recipe's oldest ingredient: **connection.**

Interlude: Enlightenment for $19.99 — The Yoga Studio Gift Shop Problem

"Can I interest you in a crystal that aligns your chakras and matches your throw pillows?"

Let's set the scene.

You've just finished a glorious 75-minute Vinyasa class.
You're glowing with sweat, inner peace, and mild dehydration.
You're proud. Grounded. Aligned.
You bow your head in Namaste.
You roll up your mat with reverence.

Then — just as you prepare to float out the door in post-Savasana bliss — you pass it.

The *altar of capitalism.*

The yoga studio gift shop.

Suddenly You're Not "Complete"

It begins innocently enough.

"Oh look," you say, "a little incense."

Next to the incense? A hand-poured candle called **'Shanti Spice Moon.'**
Next to the candle? A brass Ganesh statue with a sticker: *'Obstacles? Not today, karmic cowboy.'*

Before you know it, you're holding:

- A singing bowl
- A gratitude journal made of vegan bark
- A $92 mala made from "responsibly sourced volcanic patience stones"

The person behind the desk, dressed in linen and serenity, smiles and says:

"Those are *charged* under a Scorpio moon by an elder in Joshua Tree."

Suddenly, your yoga practice feels incomplete without them.

How Did We Get Here?

It's a tale as old as time — or at least as old as Lululemon:

Spiritual practices enter a new culture...
People resonate...
The demand for tools increases...
And then someone says, "Wait... can we *brand* this?"

And thus, **inner peace became a shelf item.**

Now don't get me wrong — I love a good candle.

But somewhere between the "chakra teas" and the $65 tie-dyed yoga strap "blessed by dolphins," the whole thing starts to feel... a bit much.

When Yoga Meets Retail Therapy

Let's play a little game called "Spiritual Tool or Etsy Prank?"

(Answers at the end.)

1. Rose quartz-infused kombucha.
2. Yoga mat bag with built-in diffuser.
3. Himalayan salt lamp shaped like Buddha riding a unicorn.
4. Limited-edition "enlightenment potion" in a glass vial with gold flakes.

(If you guessed "all of the above," you'd sadly be correct.)

Humor Break: Stuff I've Almost Bought in a Studio Gift Shop

- A crystal "third-eye stimulator" that looked suspiciously like a forehead plunger.
- An "energy wand" that resembled a glue stick.
- A shirt that said **"I bend so I don't break"** (but the font was Comic Sans — unforgivable).
- A subscription box for **spiritual snacks**. (Still not sure what those were. Probably almonds wearing mala beads.)

Why We Buy Stuff After Yoga (Science Edition)

Turns out there's psychology behind this madness.

According to studies on "post-ritual vulnerability," people are more likely to make impulse purchases immediately after emotionally or spiritually intense experiences.

Why?

Because we:

1. Feel open and expansive
2. Have temporarily lowered defenses
3. Want to **extend** the feeling we just had
4. Are in a trance-like daze from breathwork and delayed lunch

So when a handcrafted $48 palo santo bundle is positioned next to a chalkboard that reads "You Are Enough (but this bracelet helps)," it feels like fate.

Is It Bad to Buy Spiritual Stuff?

Not at all. Tools can be beautiful, meaningful, and even effective.

A candle lit with intention can be a **ritual**.

A crystal that reminds you to breathe? That's **useful magic**.

The problem isn't the stuff.

The problem is thinking the stuff *is* the practice.

You don't need:

- A $200 yoga mat made of aerated moonstone
- An eye pillow stuffed with labradorite tears
- A digital app that chants mantras in six languages (but charges monthly)

You need presence. Breath. Willingness.

And maybe a decent mat that doesn't smell like recycled gym socks. (We're not monsters.)

How to Tell If You're Buying a Tool or a Distraction

Ask yourself:

"Would this still have meaning if no one saw me use it?"

If the answer is yes — great.

If the answer is "only if I post it to Instagram with #GoddessVibes"— maybe pause.

Because spiritual consumerism can sneakily become spiritual *performance.*

And while yoga welcomes everyone, the real practice happens **inward**, not in the mirror or the merch aisle.

The Irony Is Ancient

You know who'd be side-eyeing the studio gift shop?

Patanjali.

Our dear Yoga Sūtra sage, sitting cross-legged somewhere in the cosmos, watching us charge crystals with moonlight while overcharging our credit cards.

Patanjali was big on **non-attachment** — *aparigraha*, the practice of letting go of possessions, clinging, and... well, compulsive candle-buying.

He might gently ask:

"Are you purifying your soul or just your living room?"

A fair question, Patanjali.

We'll get back to you after we check if this incense "balances our fire dosha."

How to Ground Spiritual Practice in a Consumer Culture

1. **Ritual over Retail.**

   Light a candle? Beautiful. Think it'll save your life? Maybe rethink.

2. **Invest in Teachers, Not Trinkets.**

   A great class, book, or training lasts longer than a gemstone water bottle.

3. **Practice Before You Purchase.**

   Ask: "Have I done yoga today, or just yoga-adjacent shopping?"

4. **Check for Ego in Enlightenment.**

   If your new meditation pillow is just so you can feel superior at sangha... maybe just sit on a regular cushion and reflect on that.

5. **Laugh at It All.**

   The moment you can laugh at your spiritual materialism is the moment you become immune to it.

Campfire Takeaway

There's nothing wrong with liking beautiful things.

There's nothing wrong with buying a singing bowl or a shirt that says "Zen AF."

But remember this:

Enlightenment isn't for sale.

It's not packaged.
It's not scented with jasmine.
It doesn't come with free shipping.

It comes when you *don't need anything extra to feel whole.*

Not the mat.
Not the leggings.
Not even the Himalayan salt bath infused with mantras whispered by artisanal monks.

It comes when you lie down, breathe, and realize:

"This moment — breath, body, being — is enough."

And if you still want the candle afterward?

Fine. Just don't forget to actually light it.

Chapter 12: Yoga for the Overthinker — Meditation That Moves

"If I could just stop thinking... about thinking... then I'd be perfect. Right?"

Meet the Mind: Loud, Loyal, and Endlessly Annoying

Let's start with a scene we've all lived:

You're in yoga class.

The lights are dim. The music is soft. The teacher says in their best "spiritual sleep podcast" voice:

"Clear your mind. Be present."

And instantly, your brain goes:

- "Did I lock the door?"
- "I should meal prep more."
- "What's my yoga mat made of? Why does it smell like almonds?"
- "Are my feet emotionally aligned?"

Congratulations! You're an overthinker. And you're not alone.

In fact, modern life practically breeds overthinkers. We scroll, multitask, analyze, and spiral — often before breakfast. Our minds are trained to never shut up, especially when asked nicely.

Science Says: The Brain's a Busy-Body

According to neuroscience, the average person has around 6,000+ thoughts a day. And for those of us who identify as "cognitive gymnasts," it can feel like 6,000 thoughts per hour.

What's to blame?

Mostly, the Default Mode Network — a web of brain regions responsible for:

- Self-reflection
- Mental time travel
- Daydreaming
- Replaying arguments from 2017

The DMN is your internal monologue on loop — and while it's vital for identity and memory, it's also what fuels that mental white noise we mistake for our actual self.

Here's the kicker:

The DMN goes quiet during mindful movement.

Yes. You can't outthink the mind.
But you can outflow it.

Vinyasa: Meditation in Motion (with Bonus Sweating)

This is why Vinyasa Yoga is the overthinker's best friend.

You're too focused on breathing, balancing, reaching, and not falling into your neighbor to spiral into a three-act anxiety narrative about that email you haven't answered.

That's the magic of **moving meditation**.

While still meditation asks the mind to sit down and behave (spoiler: it won't), Vinyasa says:

"Okay, mind. You like doing things? Fine. Let's *do* presence."

Every inhale and exhale becomes a metronome for awareness.
Each pose is a bookmark — anchoring you to *now*.

You don't have to fight your thoughts.
You just have to give them something better to do.

Humor Break: How Overthinkers Meditate

- "Be present." → Starts a grocery list.
- "Focus on your breath." → Hyper-fixates on whether breathing is weird.
- "Let thoughts go." → Compulsively chases each one like it's a lost puppy.
- "No judgment." → Judges self for judging. Then judges the judgment.
- "Find inner peace." → Googles "What does inner peace even *feel* like?"

Redefining Meditation (So It Doesn't Feel Like Failure)

Here's the good news:

You don't need to "empty your mind" to meditate.

In fact, the original yogic texts — like the Yoga Sūtras of Patañjali — don't ask you to stop thinking. They ask you to still the fluctuations of the mind (*chitta vritti nirodhah*).

Stillness doesn't mean silence.
It means non-reactivity.

You're allowed to think. You just don't have to follow every thought down a rabbit hole, build it a house, and furnish it with anxiety.

Movement-Based Mindfulness Techniques (That Actually Work)

Let's get practical. Here are five mind-taming tricks that pair beautifully with your yoga practice:

1. The One-Word Anchor

Choose a word — any word — and sync it with your breath.
Example:

- Inhale: "Here"
- Exhale: "Now"

Or...

- Inhale: "Calm"
- Exhale: "Down"

Or, if you're in a spicy mood:

- Inhale: "Why"
- Exhale: "Me"

The point isn't perfection. It's returning. Over and over.

2. Sensory Name-It Game

During a pose, silently label:

- What you see
- What you hear
- What you feel (inside and outside)

You're not fixing — you're witnessing.
And witnessing without judgment = *ta-da!* You're meditating.

3. Micro-Movement Mantras

As you transition between poses, repeat a phrase internally:

- "I am here."
- "This is enough."
- "Feet are weird, but I accept them."

Over time, these phrases become familiar trails through your inner forest.

4. "Notice and Nod" Method

When thoughts arise — and they will — just mentally say:

"Ah, thinking."
And gently return to breath.

It's not rejection. It's redirection.
Like a toddler trying to eat sand — you lovingly guide them away without yelling.

5. Savasana Storytime

Turn your final rest pose into a story:

- Imagine your breath as waves.
- Your body as a beach.
- Thoughts as seagulls. (They come. They go. Occasionally, they poop.)

Use creative metaphors to engage your mind without giving it the car keys.

Backed by Brains: What the Research Shows

In a 2019 study by the *Journal of Neuroscience*, participants who practiced mindful movement (like yoga) for 8 weeks showed:

- Decreased activity in the DMN
- Increased gray matter in areas linked to emotion regulation and awareness
- Improved attention span (aka, the ability to not panic every time the phone buzzes)

Vinyasa Yoga has also been shown to reduce cortisol (the stress hormone) and increase GABA (a neurotransmitter that helps you chill without wine).

So yes — yoga physically rewires your anxious, overachieving brain.

Myth-Busting: "Real Meditation Happens in Silence"

This one's for the purists who say if you're not sitting cross-legged in a Himalayan cave for 10 days in noble silence, you're not *really* meditating.

To them, we say:

- Walking is meditation.
- Folding laundry can be meditation.
- Dancing in your kitchen while breathing consciously? Totally meditation.

Stillness isn't about body posture.

It's about mental posture — and that can be found in Tree Pose *or* while wobbling during Half Moon wondering if your butt is aligned with the cosmos.

Campfire Takeaway

Overthinking isn't your enemy — it's just your mind trying to protect you with words, plans, and reruns of awkward moments.

But you don't have to obey every mental notification.

When you show up on the mat, link breath to movement, and redirect your attention from thought to sensation — even once — you've entered the practice of moving meditation.

You, my dear reader, are the snow globe.
The thoughts are snowflakes.
And yoga?

It's the gentle setting down that lets the flakes settle — not vanish, but soften — revealing the peaceful little village underneath.

So overthink all you want.
Just don't forget to breathe.
And maybe, just maybe, try thinking on purpose next time.

That's the new yoga.

Chapter 13: The Neuroscience of Flow — What Your Brain Is Doing While You Pretend to Breathe Calmly

"Yoga brain" is real. So is accidentally zoning out during Warrior II and thinking about tacos.

What Is Flow, and Can I Get It in a Bottle?

If you've ever lost track of time while doing something — writing, painting, surfing, knitting aggressively — then congratulations, you've experienced flow.

Psychologist Mihaly Csikszentmihalyi (yes, that's his real name; no, I can't say it without pulling a mental hamstring) defined flow as:

"A state of optimal experience where one is fully immersed in a feeling of energized focus, full involvement, and enjoyment in the process of the activity."

Basically, flow is when:

- You stop thinking about yourself
- Time gets weird
- You forget to check your phone (gasp)
- You don't even realize you're hungry until it's over
- And somehow, everything just… *clicks*

Now imagine applying that to yoga.

Flow in Vinyasa isn't just a poetic metaphor — it's a neurological event.

But before we get there, we need to meet the cast of characters inside your head.

Meet the Brain Team

Let's take a quick tour of your noggin, yoga edition:

- **Prefrontal Cortex**: The CEO. Responsible for planning, decision-making, and questioning whether you're doing that pose right. (Spoiler: you are.)
- **Default Mode Network (DMN)**: The daydreamer. Loves overthinking, reminiscing, and narrating your life like it's a moody indie film.
- **Amygdala**: Your internal fire alarm. Constantly scanning for saber-toothed tigers or aggressive yoga mats.
- **Insula**: The feeler. Keeps track of internal body sensations — like the sudden realization that you have hips.
- **Cerebellum**: The graceful mover. Coordinates balance, movement, and not falling over in Half Moon.

Now, under normal circumstances, these regions chat constantly — kind of like a chaotic Zoom meeting where nobody's muted and the Wi-Fi is sketchy.

But during flow, something magical happens.

Flow Brain: The Default Mode Network Takes a Nap

When you're in flow:

- Your prefrontal cortex powers down. (No more "Am I doing this right?")
- Your DMN quiets. (No more flashbacks to middle school.)

- Your amygdala chills out. (Less "fight or flight," more "fold and breathe.")
- The insula lights up. (You become deeply aware of body and breath.)
- Dopamine and norepinephrine rise. (You feel good and alert.)
- Time perception gets weird. (Was that five minutes or five decades?)

It's like your brain's usual chatter goes to voicemail, and the body — glorious, messy, breathing body — gets to drive for once.

Research Says: Yoga Induces Flow

Science time!

Multiple studies (see: Harvard Medical School, National Institutes of Health) have shown that yoga:

- Increases GABA (gamma-aminobutyric acid), which reduces anxiety
- Improves interoception (the ability to feel what's happening inside)
- Enhances alpha brainwaves, associated with relaxed alertness
- And reduces activity in the Default Mode Network, aka the Overthinking Olympics

Translation:

Practicing yoga literally changes your brain so you can focus, feel better, and not mentally spiral every time your boss emails "Can we chat?"

Flow isn't a fluke.
It's a *state* you can train.
And yoga — especially breath-based, intentional Vinyasa — is one of the most powerful ways to get there.

How Flow Shows Up on the Mat

Here's what flow might feel like in your yoga practice:

- You're moving, breathing, and the sequence feels like music.
- You're not self-conscious, but deeply embodied.
- The teacher cues "inhale, reach" — and you're already there.
- Your brain isn't narrating — it's witnessing.
- Savasana sneaks up like a ninja, and you think, "Wait, that was an hour?"

This isn't fantasy. This is neurological alignment with the present moment.

You're no longer thinking your way through practice — you're *living* it.

And unlike a runner's high, you don't need a marathon to get there. Just a mat, a breath, and a willingness to surrender your need to "nail it."

Humor Break: Signs You're Almost in Flow, But Not Quite

- You forget what pose you're in and end up inventing "Twisted Dolphin Flamingo."
- The teacher says "release tension," and you wonder if that includes your in-laws.
- You're so immersed you forget which limb is left. (Bonus points if you collapse and laugh.)
- You reach meditative bliss — until someone farts in Happy Baby and you lose it.

Flow isn't always elegant. Sometimes it's messy. But when it clicks? Ohhh, baby.

But What If I Can't Get Into Flow?

Let's get real: Not every yoga practice feels flowy.

Sometimes you're just tired.
Sometimes your mat is squeaky.
Sometimes your neighbor is breathing like Darth Vader.

That's okay.

Flow isn't a goal. It's a side effect.

It emerges when the following ingredients align:

1. **Challenge meets skill.**

    Too easy = boredom. Too hard = panic. Just right = immersion.

2. **Clear structure.**

    Vinyasa's sequences give your mind a rhythm to follow.

3. **Immediate feedback.**

    Breath too short? You feel it. Balance lost? Your body tells you.

4. **Focused attention.**

    The more your mind tunes into the moment, the less space there is

    for wandering.

Flow Off the Mat

Now here's where things get fun.

Practicing flow on the mat teaches you how to access it **off** the mat:

*   Cooking dinner while totally immersed in chopping garlic

- Walking through the woods and suddenly feeling time dissolve
- Deeply engaged in a conversation or project without checking your phone every 47 seconds

Yoga rewires your brain not just for *mat-magic*, but for everyday presence.

Campfire Takeaway

Flow is not reserved for elite athletes or monk-level meditators. It's not about achieving bliss or floating six inches above your mat.

Flow is what happens when your body, breath, and attention finally stop fighting — and start dancing.

And Vinyasa Yoga, done with intention and curiosity, is your dance floor.

You won't find flow in forcing a pose.
You'll find it in losing yourself inside the breath.

So next time you show up on your mat, let the brain rest. Let the breath lead. And if your inner narrator pipes up with "Are we doing this right?" — smile and say:

"Shhh. We're flowing now."

Chapter 14: Off the Mat and Into the Pub — Karma Yoga in Daily Life

"Because what good is inner peace if it disappears the second someone steals your parking spot?"

The Yoga Most People Don't Teach in Class

Let's start with a small heresy:

The real yoga test isn't how long you can hold Crow Pose.

It's how calmly you can sit in traffic when someone cuts you off and gives *you* the finger.

Or when your toddler lovingly smears hummus on the dog.

Or when your friend cancels on you (again) with the world's worst excuse: "My aura felt off."

This is the moment Karma Yoga strolls in, takes off its sandals, and says:

"Hey buddy, this is the yoga you *actually* signed up for."

Karma Yoga is the yoga of action.

It's not about what happens on your mat — it's about how you live when you're not on it.

Wait... What Is Karma Yoga, Really?

Let's time travel back to the Bhagavad Gītā, yoga's ancient mic-drop text.

The hero, Arjuna, is standing on a battlefield having a full-blown existential meltdown. He's supposed to go to war, but he's like,

111

"This feels morally complicated. Maybe I'll just sit here and vibe instead."

Enter Lord Krishna, disguised as his charioteer (plot twist: he's also an avatar of Vishnu — just your average Uber driver/god). Krishna delivers this classic line:

"You have a right to the work, but not to the fruits of the work."

Translation?

Do the thing.
Do it with your full heart.
But let go of the outcome.

That's Karma Yoga.

Modern Karma Yoga: Illustrated via Mildly Traumatizing Life Situations

1. You Clean the Kitchen. Your Roommate Destroys It in 4 Minutes.

Karma Yoga says: Do the dishes anyway. Not for applause. Not for praise. Not even for Instagram.
Just… because it's the right thing.

2. You're in Line at the Coffee Shop. Someone Cuts. Loudly. Rudely. Smelling of Axe Body Spray.

Karma Yoga says: You can speak up, sure — but do it from a place of clarity, not rage. (And then let it go. With dignity. And a large oat milk latte.)

3. You Meditate Every Day for a Month. Still Anxious. Still Snapping at Your Partner.

Karma Yoga says: That's okay. The point isn't instant transformation. It's staying in the game without demanding gold stars for effort.

The Science of "Selfless Action"

Neuroscience is catching up with the Bhagavad Gītā (about 2,000 years late, but we'll allow it).

Research on pro-social behavior — actions that benefit others without expectation — shows:

- Increases in dopamine and oxytocin (the feel-good, love-hormone cocktail)
- Decreases in stress-related cortisol
- Enhanced sense of purpose and well-being

In short, when you serve without attachment, **you feel better**, people like you more, and your nervous system throws you a party.

It's almost like ancient yogis… knew things?

Humor Break: Karma Yoga in Everyday Places

Karma Yoga at the Grocery Store

- Cart stuck.
- Kid screaming.
- Self-checkout says "Unexpected Item in Bagging Area."
  You smile. Help someone lift a watermelon. Breathe.
  Win.

Karma Yoga at Family Dinner

- Uncle starts ranting about conspiracy theories.
- Your job: Don't erupt. Just pass the mashed potatoes with grace.
  Victory.

Karma Yoga in Text Threads

- Someone misreads your message and gets snippy.
- You resist the urge to respond with a passive-aggressive GIF.
  You respond with clarity. Or not at all.
  Nirvana.

Work as Worship (No, Seriously)

The Gītā says **every action**, when done with mindfulness and no clinging, becomes sacred.

That means:

- Making spreadsheets = yoga
- Parenting a tantruming 3-year-old = yoga
- Folding laundry without resentment = *advanced* yoga
- Picking up dog poop at 6am = enlightenment, basically

This isn't about being a doormat.
It's about being unshakable in purpose and soft in ego.

Karma Yoga isn't passive. It's powerful.
It's presence in action.
It's devotion with dish gloves on.

The Big Trap: "If I Do Good, Good Things Should Happen... Right?"

Ah. The secret fantasy of the spiritually ambitious.

"I helped five people cross the street. Where's my cosmic reward?"

But Karma Yoga laughs gently and says:

"You do it because it needs doing.
You let go of the scoreboard.
That *is* the reward."

This is yoga as adulthood.
Yoga as reality.
Yoga as surrender-with-a-spine.

It's not about floating above suffering.
It's about meeting life fully — messy, unpredictable, hilarious — with equanimity.

Karma Yoga On and Off the Mat

On the mat:

- You move without chasing a perfect pose.
- You breathe without berating your wandering mind.
- You return, again and again, without demanding applause.

Off the mat:

- You show up at work.
- You love your people.
- You empty the dishwasher.
- You recycle, even when it's confusing.

Not because someone's watching.
But because *you are*.

Campfire Takeaway

We've been conditioned to chase gold stars — in school, in jobs, in yoga classes where we're just *dying* to be noticed in that flawless crow pose.

But Karma Yoga hands you a steaming mug of tea and says:

"Do your work.
Give your heart.
Let go of what comes next."

It's not sexy.
It won't go viral on TikTok.
But it will **free your soul** from the tyranny of "what do I get?"

Because when you serve without clinging —
When you flow without grabbing —
When you live from love, not outcome —

That's when yoga leaves the studio
and walks with you into real life.

Yes, even into the pub.
Especially into the pub.

Because if you can breathe mindfully while someone rants about politics over fries…

Congratulations. You are now a master yogi.

Chapter 15: Final Savasana — The Ultimate Pose and the Ultimate Letting Go

"Lie down like you've got nothing to prove and nowhere to be — because for once, it's true."

The Yoga Pose Most People Nail

Let's be honest: most people's *favorite* yoga pose is **Savasana** — a Sanskrit word that means "corpse pose," which is possibly the most metal name for something that involves lying on your back and doing absolutely nothing.

And yet...
It's the hardest pose of all.

Because when you're truly still — not napping, not fidgeting, not secretly planning dinner — you come face to face with your **unfiltered self**.

And the question arises:

"Can I just *be* without trying to become something else?"

Welcome to the final exhale. The grand finale. The moment every yoga practice builds toward:

Letting go.

Why Is It Called Corpse Pose, Though?

It's not just poetic.

Savasana is called "corpse pose" because it symbolizes ego death — the temporary surrender of identity, control, and attachment.

117

You lie down as your "doer" self — the one who tweaks, plans, poses, performs — and in those five or ten minutes of deep stillness, you release all striving.

You become, for a moment, no one and everything.

No goals. No effort. Just breath and presence and the ground holding you.

It's your daily dress rehearsal for surrender.
For trusting the process.
For being enough.

And yes — symbolically, it's a micro-practice for the ultimate letting go: death.

But we'll get to that. After one more joke, probably.

Humor Break: How People *Actually* Do Savasana

- One person lies there like a serene forest elf.
- One person forgets where they are and starts softly snoring.
- One guy scratches his nose 17 times.
- Someone is clearly trying not to fart.
- You? You're wondering if it's too early to get tacos. And yet — *somehow* — this is yoga at its deepest.

The Nervous System's Greatest Hits: Rest & Digest

Here's what your body's doing while you're "just lying there":

- Activating the parasympathetic nervous system — your body's rest-and-digest mode.
- Lowering cortisol and blood pressure.

118

- Balancing your heart rate variability, which is a fancy way of saying your body is learning to chill better.
- Encouraging deep integration of the physical, mental, and emotional layers you've moved through in class.

Savasana is not a throwaway.

It's the moment when all the movement and breathwork settle into the body's archive — becoming part of who you are, not just what you did.

It's like hitting "Save As" on your practice.

Neurologically Speaking: The Power of Stillness

Science time!

Researchers have found that deep rest states — like those achieved in Savasana or non-sleep deep rest (NSDR) techniques — activate the default mode network (the part of the brain responsible for self-awareness and memory), but in a *healed*, regulated way.

Instead of spiraling, your brain begins to reorganize and integrate.

Translation:

Your mind gets smarter by resting.
Your body becomes more stable.
Your emotional system learns safety.

And you didn't even have to lift a dumbbell.

You just had to lie down and *not* check your phone for 10 minutes.

Savasana and the Spiritual Mic Drop

Every yoga tradition, from Hatha to Tantra to Vedanta, honors Savasana as sacred.

Why?

Because it's the symbolic surrender of the small self.

It says:

- I am not my to-do list.
- I am not my bank balance or my Instagram bio.
- I am not my productivity.
- I am not even my yoga practice.

I am breath.
I am space.
I am alive — right now — and that is *enough*.

This is where yoga becomes less about "doing" and more about undoing.

Letting go of control.
Letting go of expectation.
Letting go of needing to fix or improve anything in this moment.

That's liberation.

Okay But... Death?

Yes, Savasana points gently (but unavoidably) toward **death** — not in a morbid way, but in a freeing way.

Every time you lie down in stillness, you practice releasing your identity, your tension, your mental grip on "being someone."

And what's left?

Awareness. Spaciousness. Connection.

Ironically, it's in pretending to be a corpse that we *feel most alive*.

Yoga doesn't deny death.
It includes it — as part of the rhythm of breath, cycles, energy.
Inhale: Life.
Exhale: Letting go.

This isn't about being fearless.
It's about being honest — and present — with what is.

Even if what is… is unknown.

How to *Actually* Do Savasana (Without Fidgeting or Faking It)

1. Get Comfy.

Blanket? Yes. Eye pillow? Absolutely. Yoga burrito? Highly recommended.

2. Set an Intention — Then Let It Go.

Like planting a seed and walking away. Trust the soil.

3. Follow the Breath Like a Lazy River.

Don't force it. Just ride it.

4. Notice Thoughts Like Weather.

They pass. You stay.

5. When You Want to Get Up — Stay.

That's usually when the real Savasana begins.

6. When You Rise, Rise Gently.

Like you're re-entering the world as a slightly more awake human being.

Everyday Savasana: Off the Mat, Into the Mess

You can practice Savasana **anywhere**:

- On your couch after a long day.
- In your parked car before going into a meeting.
- Sitting at your kitchen table, sipping tea, watching rain fall.

The pose isn't the point.

It's the **willingness to pause**, breathe, and remember who you are without doing anything.

It's choosing presence over productivity.
Stillness over scrambling.
Being over becoming.

Campfire Takeaway

If Vinyasa is the story,
and breath is the rhythm,
and movement is the language,
then Savasana is the final page, the soft exhale, the sacred silence between heartbeats.

You've earned it.

Lie down.
Let go.
Feel the ground beneath you, supporting everything you are.

And know this:

You are not here to conquer your body, prove your worth, or perfect a pose.
You are here to remember.
And in Savasana — you finally do.

Interlude: Confessions of a Yoga Class Addict (or, How I Accidentally Joined a Cult of Elastic Pants)

Let's begin with a confession.

I didn't mean to become a yoga person.

I signed up for my first Vinyasa class because I thought it was a low-impact way to get in shape. "Just stretching," I told myself. "Some gentle breathing. Maybe a candle."

Forty-five minutes later, I was upside down, sweating from my *eyelashes*, trying not to collapse into a puddle of existential dread while the teacher whispered things like "Find your truth" and "Breathe into your spleen."

At one point I think I wept silently in Pigeon Pose. No one told me my hip flexors were hiding repressed childhood trauma.

So yeah. One class in and I was hooked.

Not on the poses. Not on the burn.
But on the absurdity of it all.

Because yoga, friends — yoga is weird.

A Brief Timeline of a Typical Yoga Class (for Normal Humans)

Minute 0–5: Arrival.

You walk into the studio. It's quiet. Serene. Smells vaguely like lavender

125

and a sweaty sock. The room is full of people silently stretching like ancient cats.

You try to look casual. Your mat unrolls with a violent *thwack*. Everyone turns. You're now "that guy."

Minute 6–15: Warming Up.

Some cat-cows. Some gentle lunges. You feel confident. Loose. Maybe you *are* a natural yogi.

Minute 16–30: The Struggle Begins.

Warrior II becomes Warrior Why. The teacher says "Engage your core," and you wonder if you've *ever* had a core. You lock eyes with a stranger in Downward Dog and see your shared soul exhaustion reflected back.

Minute 31–45: Ego Death.

The teacher introduces Crow Pose. You try. You fall. You pretend it was on purpose. Your body shakes like a newborn giraffe. Someone farts. You try not to laugh. You remember you are a speck of dust in an infinite cosmos.

Minute 46–60: Savasana.

You lie on your back like a toastless avocado. You melt. You dissolve. You forget your name. The teacher rings a singing bowl. You ascend briefly into the astral plane. Then someone drops their water bottle and you're yanked back to Earth.

Class over.

The Yoga Persona Starter Pack

By Month 2, you've acquired:

- 1 pair of pants that cost more than your rent
- A mat made from recycled unicorn tears
- A mala bead necklace you don't know how to use
- An increasing suspicion that your yoga teacher is a wizard
- A collection of tote bags with slogans like:
    - "Let That Sh*t Go"
    - "I'm Just Here for Savasana"
    - "Peace, Love, and Hip Openers (Please Send Help)"

Things I Still Don't Understand About Yoga Culture

- Why is everyone suddenly obsessed with turmeric?
- Who is "this Patanjali guy" and why is he judging my alignment?
- Why does one pose make me feel like Beyoncé and another like I'm folding a patio chair with my spine?

And most importantly:

Why do I keep coming back?

Unexpected Side Effects of Frequent Yoga

- You begin saying "Namaste" at inappropriate times. (Barista hands you coffee? "Namaste.")
- You accidentally *breathe through* minor inconveniences.
- You start prefacing arguments with, "From a heart-centered place…"
- You notice your emotions hiding in your **hips**, of all places.

- You catch yourself watching a leaf fall and whisper, "That's the lesson."

It's a slippery slope.

The Weirdest Class I Ever Took

Let me tell you about the time I signed up for something called "Yogic Primal Flow."

The class began with animal noises.

I'm not joking.

There were howls. Grunts. One woman shrieked like a hawk in labor. We were told to "release our inner mammal."

Then we did something called "shamanic rolling," which looked like interpretive flopping.

At one point I made eye contact with a man in full Lion's Breath, and we both instantly regretted it.

I left that class confused, sore, and somehow… emotionally free?

Yoga's weird. But weird is healing.

Things I've Whispered to Myself in Class

- "No one saw that fall. No one saw that fall."
- "Is this pose *supposed* to make my elbow feel like it's trying to speak Latin?"
- "This must be what enlightenment feels like… Oh wait, I left my car windows down."

- "That guy's breath sounds like Darth Vader on a rowing machine."
- "Please, yoga gods, don't let the teacher say handstand."

The Great Cosmic Joke

After years of yoga classes, workshops, philosophy talks, breathwork sessions, and one regrettable cacao ceremony, here's the big lesson I've learned:

It's all a game. A sacred, sweaty, occasionally ridiculous game.

You come in thinking you'll get flexible.
You leave wondering who you *really* are.
And somewhere along the way, you stop caring whether your hamstrings ever "open up" and start noticing when your heart does.

Yoga gives you tools to deal with life's curveballs.

But more than that, it teaches you that:

- Falling is normal.
- Breathing helps.
- Lying on the floor is a legitimate spiritual practice.
- And sometimes the most powerful mantra is "whatever."

Campfire Takeaway

So here's to the yoga misfits.
The ones who fall out of poses and laugh.
The ones who come for fitness and stay for philosophy.
The ones who don't quite belong — but somehow *do*.

If you've ever felt weird in a yoga class, you're not alone.
If you've ever questioned whether you're "doing it right," you probably are.
And if you've ever lain in Savasana and thought, "I love this weird, beautiful, bendy cult of calm," welcome.

You're one of us now.

Namaste, nerds.
Let's go get a smoothie.

Bibliography

Primary Yogic Texts & Translations

- Bryant, Edwin F. *The Yoga Sūtras of Patañjali: A New Edition, Translation, and Commentary.* North Point Press, 2009.

- Easwaran, Eknath. *The Bhagavad Gita.* Nilgiri Press, 2007.

- Swami Satchidananda. *The Yoga Sutras of Patanjali: Commentary.* Integral Yoga Publications, 2012.

- Feuerstein, Georg. *The Yoga Tradition: Its History, Literature, Philosophy and Practice.* Hohm Press, 2001.

- Mallinson, James, and Singleton, Mark. *Roots of Yoga.* Penguin Classics, 2017.

Modern Interpretations and Commentaries

- Iyengar, B.K.S. *Light on Yoga.* Schocken Books, 1979.

- Desikachar, T.K.V. *The Heart of Yoga: Developing a Personal Practice.* Inner Traditions International, 1995.

- Jois, Pattabhi. *Yoga Mala.* North Point Press, 2002.

- Saraswati, Swami Satyananda. *Asana Pranayama Mudra Bandha.* Bihar School of Yoga, 2008.

- Sivananda Yoga Vedanta Centre. *The Sivananda Companion to Yoga.* Fireside, 1983.

Neuroscience, Psychology & Health Research

- Siegel, Daniel J. *The Mindful Brain.* W.W. Norton & Company, 2007.

- Goleman, Daniel, and Davidson, Richard. *Altered Traits: Science Reveals How Meditation Changes Your Mind, Brain, and Body.* Avery, 2017.

- Rossi, Ernest Lawrence. *The Psychobiology of Mind-Body Healing.* Norton, 1993.

- van der Kolk, Bessel. *The Body Keeps the Score.* Penguin Books, 2014.

- Lazar, Sara W., et al. "Meditation experience is associated with increased cortical thickness." *Neuroreport*, 2005.

Humor, Creativity & Cultural Commentary

- Lamott, Anne. *Bird by Bird: Some Instructions on Writing and Life.* Anchor Books, 1995.

- Gilbert, Elizabeth. *Big Magic: Creative Living Beyond Fear.* Riverhead Books, 2015.

- McGraw, Phil. *Self Matters: Creating Your Life from the Inside Out.* Free Press, 2001.

Miscellaneous Sources & Influences

- Kripalu Center for Yoga & Health – Workshop Materials and Teaching Manuals.

- Yoga Journal archives (various issues, 2000–2022).

- Podcast: "Yoga is Dead" by Tejal Patel and Jesal Parikh – Selected episodes on yoga history, culture, and appropriation.

- Lectures from the Himalayan Institute and Yoga International (transcripts and study notes).

- Personal communications with yoga educators and Ayurvedic practitioners (names anonymized for privacy).

- User-provided research report: *Exploring Traditional Vinyasa Yoga Philosophy* (uploaded and reviewed internally).

Note: This bibliography combines traditional sources with modern interpretations and relevant scientific research to support the tone, teachings, and humor-laced insights of the book.

Glossary of Terms from Stillness in Motion: The Campfire Guide to Traditional Vinyasa Yoga

Abhyāsa

"Practice."
The consistent, dedicated effort toward steadying the mind. Think of it as mental flossing — daily, necessary, not always glamorous.

Āsana

"Seat" or "posture."
Commonly used to refer to yoga poses. Traditionally, it referred to the seated posture for meditation. Now it includes everything from Downward Dog to "I Regret This Lunge."

Bandha

"Lock" or "seal."
Energetic locks used to control and direct prāṇa in the body. Think of them like the valves in your inner plumbing system: subtle, powerful, and occasionally mysterious.

Bhagavad Gītā

A sacred Hindu scripture that's basically a conversation between a warrior (Arjuna) having an existential meltdown and his divine charioteer (Krishna), who's like a life coach meets the universe.

Chakra

"Wheel" or "disk."
Seven (main) energy centers along the spine, each associated with physical, emotional, and spiritual functions. Also: a great way to justify mood swings.

Citta

"Mind-stuff" or "consciousness."
The full field of mental activity — thoughts, feelings, memories, Netflix rewatches, etc. Yoga is the art of calming this cosmic chatter.

Drishti

"Gaze" or "focused point."
Where you look during a pose — not just physically, but energetically. Bonus: helps avoid staring awkwardly at someone else's mat.

Ego (Ahaṅkāra)

The "I" maker — the part of the mind that says, "I am this body, I am these achievements." In yoga, the ego isn't evil — it's just really loud.

Haṭha Yoga

A physical branch of yoga emphasizing postures, breath control, and purification. "Ha" (sun) + "Tha" (moon) = balance of energies. Also: where the stretchy stuff began.

Ida Nadi

The left channel of prāṇa, associated with cooling, introspection, and moon energy. If Pingala is espresso, Ida is a warm chamomile nap.

Karma Yoga

"Yoga of action."
Acting without attachment to outcomes. Doing the dishes, giving a hug, leading a revolution — all can be Karma Yoga with the right mindset.

Krama

"Sequence" or "step-by-step progression."
Key to Vinyasa Krama — the idea that everything unfolds with intelligence, like a well-layered lasagna (which, yes, we reference often).

Kṛṣṇa

The divine charioteer in the Bhagavad Gītā. Also known as the ultimate spiritual wingman. Dispenses cosmic truth mid-battle without breaking a sweat.

Mudrā

"Gesture" or "seal."
Hand positions (and sometimes full-body gestures) that direct energy flow. Also makes you look *extremely* intentional on Instagram.

Nāḍī

Subtle energy channel through which prāṇa flows. There are said to be 72,000 in the human body. (Good luck finding them on a map.)

Patañjali

Ancient sage and compiler of the *Yoga Sūtras*. Kind of like the Steve Jobs of classical yoga — less turtlenecks, more transcendence.

Pingalā Nadi

The right channel of prāṇa, linked with heat, activity, and sun energy. The coffee to Ida's tea.

Prāṇa

"Life force."
Not just breath — the vital energy that animates you. Think of it as the Wi-Fi of your body: invisible, but when it's not flowing… nothing works.

Prāṇāyāma

"Breath control."
The art and science of managing prāṇa through the breath. Not holding your breath while angry — more like fine-tuning the body's energy volume.

Sādhana

"Spiritual practice."
Your daily ritual, discipline, or devotion — whether that's 6 a.m. meditation or simply not yelling at someone who cut you off in traffic.

Samādhi

"Absorption" or "blissful union."
The big cosmic exhale. The deepest state of meditative awareness where self dissolves. Not available in stores.

Sanskrit

Ancient language of yoga and the Vedas. Beautiful, poetic, and occasionally impossible to pronounce until you're mid-chant and decide to just go for it.

Sūtra

"Thread."
A concise verse packed with meaning. Like a philosophical tweet from 2,000 years ago.

Sushumnā Nadi

The central energy channel running along the spine. Where balance, awareness, and higher states of being are said to awaken. Or, at the very least, where the tingles live.

www.ingramcontent.com/pod-product-compliance
Lightning Source LLC
Chambersburg PA
CBHW060501280326
41933CB00014B/2813

Tamas

One of the three guṇas (qualities of nature). Associated with inertia, dullness, and the feeling you get before coffee.

Tapas

"Heat" or "discipline."
The fire of willpower that keeps you showing up — even when your body says "no" and your brain says "Netflix."

Ujjāyī Breath

"Victorious breath."
That Darth Vader-ish sound you hear in Vinyasa class. Used to regulate heat, prāṇa, and sometimes emotional meltdowns.

Vairāgya

"Non-attachment."
Letting go of craving or control. Like Marie Kondo for your ego.

Vinyāsa

"To place in a special way."
The art of linking movement with breath. Not just flailing — intentional flow, one breath per movement.

Yamas & Niyamas

The ethical guidelines of yoga — like the Ten Commandments but with fewer threats and more self-inquiry.

Yoga

"Union."
Of breath and body. Mind and spirit. Self and the universe. Or, on some days, just keeping it together until Savasana.

Note: Definitions are intentionally informal, conversational, and sprinkled with humor in alignment with the tone of the book.